The Integrative Power of Cognitive Therapy

# The Integrative Power
# of Cognitive Therapy

BRAD A. ALFORD
AARON T. BECK

THE GUILFORD PRESS
New York      London

© 1997 The Guilford Press
A Division of Guilford Publications, Inc.
72 Spring Street, New York, NY 10012
www.guilford.com

Printed in the United States of America

This book is printed on acid-free paper.

Last digit is print number:   9   8   7   6   5   4   3   2

**Library of Congress Cataloging-in-Publication Data**

Alford, Brad A.
　　The integrative power of cognitive therapy / Brad A. Alford,
Aaron T. Beck.
　　　　p.　cm.
　　Includes bibliographical references and index.
　　ISBN 1-57230-171-6 (hard cover)　ISBN 1-57230-396-4 (pbk.)
　　1. Cognitive therapy.　2. Eclectic psychotherapy.　I. Beck,
Aaron T.　II. Title.
　　RC489.C63A44　1977
　　616.89′142—dc21
　　　　　　　　　　　　　　　　　　　　　　　　　96-47830
　　　　　　　　　　　　　　　　　　　　　　　　　　CIP

*To the many scholarly critics and researchers whose incisive analyses and criticisms have helped insure the continued evolution of cognitive therapy and theory, and have stimulated the preparation of this volume.*

# Acknowledgments

We would like to acknowledge the scholarly reactions and suggestions of those who read earlier versions of the manuscript, including Dave Clark, Bob Leahy, Dave Haaga, Jim Buchanan, Ruth Musetto, Tom Smith, and Geary Alford. Vince Merkel provided technical assistance in producing diskettes. Tim Cannon, Anne Baldwin, and Rob Brennan helped prepare the figures for Chapters 1 and 6. Rochelle Serwator, editor at The Guilford Press, provided many insightful observations that facilitated the timely completion of this volume. Marie Sprayberry and William Meyer, also of Guilford, helped with the production process. Finally, Cheryl and Jason Alford provided balance and perspective that allowed this volume to unfold over time, perhaps adding creativity to the writing process.

# Contents

## PART II: COGNITIVE THERAPY AND PSYCHOTHERAPY INTEGRATION

## PART III: COGNITIVE THERAPY AS INTEGRATIVE THEREAPY: EXAMPLES IN THEORY AND CLINICAL PRACTICE

# Introduction

Some time ago, it was suggested that the weight of evidence for cognitive therapy warranted its admission into the "arena of controversy," alongside behavior therapy and psychoanalysis (Beck, 1976). Since then, over 120 empirical tests (through 1993) have supported the efficacy of cognitive therapy (Hollon & Beck, 1994), and it has been applied to an impressive range of disorders.

Though the suggestion has been challenged by critics (Coyne, 1994), cognitive therapy and theory not only constitute an effective, coherent approach, but also may serve as a unifying or "integrative" paradigm for psychopathology and effective psychotherapy (Alford, 1995; Alford & Norcross, 1991; Beck, 1991a). The main purpose of this volume is to clarify issues that are judged to be most relevant to cognitive therapy as integrative therapy—that is, as a system of psychotherapy that fulfills the aims or goals of psychotherapy integration. These issues include the nature of and criteria for psychotherapy integration; theoretical coherence within the psychotherapy integration movement; the relationship of cognitive therapy to the psychotherapy integration movement; internal versus external (environmental) dimensions of cognitive theory and therapy; the nature of human consciousness and cognition; the role of interpersonal factors (including the "therapeutic relationship") in psychotherapy process and outcome; and contemporary philosophical and theoretical questions in cognitive therapy. In elaborating all of these issues, we show that it is an oversimplification to characterize cognitive therapy as focused on such narrow dimensions as behavior versus cognition; affect versus cognition; present versus past orientation; short-term versus long-term treatment; techniques versus relationship; conscious versus unconscious; automatic thoughts versus self-concept; cognitive content versus faulty cognitive processing; and attention to internal versus external or "environmental" dimensions.

Regarding the incorporation of polarities into cognitive theory and therapy, consider, for example, the British empiricist principles from which the foundations of behavior therapy emerged (Fishman & Franks, 1992). The four main philosophical principles of empiricism can be viewed as polarities, in which each thesis is in need of an antithesis in order to constitute a complete picture. In cognitive theory, such polarities are incorporated into a coherent paradigm (as discussed in Part I of this book). For example, cognitive theory suggests that (1) knowledge not only comes from experience, but also is influenced by the structure of the organism's nervous system; (2) scientific procedures not only are based upon observation, but also are shaped by the particular theory held by the experimenter who designs the procedures; (3) the mind of a child is not entirely a *tabula rasa*, but, rather, holds limited potentialities for memory, processing, and speed of calculation, as well as tendencies to attend to certain environmental stimuli and ignore others; and (4) consciousness cannot be entirely reduced to "mental chemistry," since its component parts cannot explain emergent properties (cf. Fishman & Franks, 1992, p. 161).

As the scope of cognitive theory and therapy expands, the cognitive focus of treatment evolves as well. Instead of taking a dichotomous stance, trained cognitive therapists match each disorder and patient characteristic to various points along a continuum on the dimensions described above. An increasing number of different disorders, and more severe disorders, are now treated with cognitive therapy; treatment of each disorder requires special areas of competence. In the treatment of severe problems (such as personality disorders, schizophrenia, or panic disorder), cognitive strategies and techniques cannot be implemented in the same manner as with mild to moderate clinical disorders. Cognitive therapists are now using a greater variety of treatment formats, such as group and family therapy. Treatment strategies have naturally evolved and become more specialized, compared to earlier formulations.

In this volume, we attempt to clarify certain complexities of clinical cognitive theory. We also articulate how cognitive therapy, as conceived and practiced by its developers, represents an integrating paradigm for clinical practice. In doing so, we first address a number of theoretical and metatheoretical issues that will serve to clarify the multidimensional nature of cognitive therapy (Part I); we then discuss the relationship between the psychotherapy integration movement and cognitive therapy (Part II); finally, we focus on the treatment of some complex clinical disorders as examples of the integrative nature of clinical cognitive theory and practice (Part III).

Part I is entitled "Theory and Metatheory of Cognitive Therapy," and includes three chapters. Chapter 1, "Theory," articulates how cognitive therapy is essentially the application of cognitive theory to the individual case. Cognitive theory relates the clinical disorders to specific cognitive variables, and includes a comprehensive set of principles or axioms. In this chapter, we review the early development of cognitive therapy and theory, provide a formal statement of theory, and discuss several theoretical directions and problems. Chapter 2, "Metatheory," clarifies a number of interrelated issues, including (1) the nature of theory; (2) types of "causes"; (3)

the nature of cognition; (4) cognition as a clinical–theoretical bridge; and (5) cognition and the therapeutic relationship.

Chapter 3, "Cognitive Mediation of Consequences," focuses primarily on one aspect of behavioral theory that may relate to a cognitive conceptualization—namely, temporal elements in psychopathology (i.e., how a person's actions come to be influenced by temporally remote consequences, rather than immediate consequences). A well-established psychological principle is that the *immediate* (compared to delayed) consequences of behavior exert relatively more influence on the probability of future similar responses. Consistent with experimental learning studies and clinical observation, we advance a thesis on psychopathological conflicts of consequences—that is, conflicts between short-term (immediate) and long-term (delayed) outcomes. We consider how certain theoretical constructs of cognitive therapy account for the resolution of such conflicts. In so doing, we describe an integrative theoretical perspective, in which distinct cognitive systems are seen as controlling automatic, conscious, and metacognitive processes.

Both of us have written previously regarding the integrative nature of cognitive therapy. In Part II of this volume, entitled "Cognitive Therapy and Psychotherapy Integration," we more fully develop several lines of reasoning regarding this issue. In doing so, we delineate numerous hurdles faced in combining or borrowing from the established scientific systems of psychotherapy in order to develop new integrative systems of psychotherapy (see A. A. Lazarus, 1995a). We deal simultaneously with (1) challenges by integrationists to the established systems, and (2) misconceptions regarding cognitive therapy (see Gluhoski, 1994; Weishaar, 1993, Ch. 4). In order to understand more clearly ways in which cognitive therapy is "integrative" or "unified" as a psychological therapeutic approach, we review several relevant issues and controversies within the contemporary psychotherapy integration movement.

In Chapter 4, "An Analysis of Integrative Ideology," we present a critical review of the contemporary efforts to integrate the psychotherapies. Several basic, interrelated problems in the goal of developing new integrative therapies by combining elements of "pure-form" therapies are described: (1) problems in delineating the criteria for psychotherapy integration; (2) problems in definition and specificity; (3) the reliance on surveys to understand integrative practices; (4) multiple meanings of "psychotherapy integration"; (5) the inherently political nature of psychotherapy integration; (6) failure to appreciate the virtues of scholarly debates; (7) failure to invest in scientific theories; and (8) theoretical ambiguities concerning the common-factors approach to integration. Finally, we show how cognitive therapy has addressed many of these issues by providing both a common language for clinical practice and a technically eclectic approach made coherent by cognitive theory (see A. A. Lazarus, 1995a). This chapter also addresses the nature of technical eclecticism, focusing on whether psychotherapy can really be "atheoretical." In science, the direction a discipline takes is determined by the conduct of systematic observations; however, these observations themselves are in turn products of the theoretical perspectives of scientists within a given cultural context. The distinction between cognitive therapy and technical eclecticism is addressed. Cognitive therapy is shown to emphasize both external validity (i.e., generalization) *and* theoretical coherence. In Chapter 5, "Cognitive Therapy as an Integrative Theory for Clinical Practice," we review (1) the role of theory, (2) the criteria for a scientific theory, and (3) efforts toward theoretical integration.

Part III, "Cognitive Therapy as Integrative Therapy: Examples in Theory and Clinical Practice," focuses on clinical and theoretical illustrations of the integrative nature of cognitive therapy. Panic disorder (Chapter 6) and schizophrenia and other psychotic disorders (Chapter 7) are selected for examination here; however, any number of other disorders could as readily have served as examples. In cognitive therapy of both panic disorder and psychotic disorders, a novel conceptualization and alternative meanings for symptoms are provided. Both applications are supported by a variety of data and observations, and are easily explained and taught (Beck, 1994).

Regarding the selection of panic disorder, a consensus report by the National Institute of Mental Health clearly indicated the efficacy of cognitive therapy of panic disorder, and therefore called even more strongly for a theoretical explanation of the effective treatment components (Sargent, 1990). The hypothesis of cognitivists (and most contemporary learning theorists) is that the underlying therapeutic processes are cognitive in nature. Chapter 6, "Panic Disorder: The Convergence of Conditioning and Cognitive Models," addresses this important theoretical issue in an integrative manner; namely, it presents a preliminary effort to integrate classical and operant conditioning theory with cognitive theory. Panic disorder is used to structure the discussion of the convergence between these theories. Contemporary classical conditioning models and operant formulations of panic disorder are reviewed, including panic response acquisition and maintenance. Issues in the assessment of phenomenology and the reformulation of learning principles are presented, along with how cognitive theory integrates the two basic levels of meaning (i.e., objective/public and subjective/private) and bypasses Cartesian dualism.

Turning to more severe psychopathology, Chapter 7, "Schizophrenia and Other Psychotic Disorders," devotes special attention to the theory, assessment, and treatment of these disabling conditions. These chronic disorders pose special challenges to the cognitive therapist, and their degree of complexity illustrates a particularly unified or "integrative" approach to therapy. This area represents one of the most recent areas of exploration for the application of cognitive therapy. Thus, the cognitive approach presented herein is at the "cutting edge" of available applications.

Although we hope that researchers (and graduate clinical students) will find this volume of great utility, another intended audience is clinical practitioners. Many clinicians properly feel the need for a broad (yet coherent) paradigm to guide their everyday work with patients. As we show in the pages to follow, cognitive theory provides such a paradigm. Clinical cognitive theory is shown to consist of a complex set of theoretical and metatheoretical perspectives suited to the actual demands of clinical practice. Here are some examples:

1. Cognitive therapists do not and *cannot* (according to the standard practice of cognitive therapy) exclude significant others from therapy sessions when interpersonal conflicts dominate a patient's complaints.

2. Environmental contexts cannot be ignored in those cases where a cognitive conceptualization indicates faulty personal constructions of behavioral consequences (i.e., response–reinforcement relationships), or actual conflicts of short-term versus long-term consequences within those contexts.

3. Standard cognitive therapy does not neglect the focus on unconscious issues when clinical assessment reveals early unresolved trauma in relationship to significant others.

These three examples are often incorrectly thought to lie exclusively and respectively within the domains of interpersonal, behavioral, and psychodynamic psychotherapy. On the contrary, we show in this volume that cognitive therapy provides a unifying theoretical framework within which the clinical techniques of other established, validated psychotherapeutic approaches may be properly incorporated. By assimilating proven techniques that are theoretically consistent with the cognitive perspective, cognitive therapy provides a coherent yet evolving paradigm for clinical practice.

# PART I

# THEORY AND METATHEORY
# OF COGNITIVE THERAPY

# CHAPTER ONE

# Theory

Cognitive theory articulates the manner in which cognitive processes are implicated in psychopathology and in effective psychotherapy. Although the "biopsychosocial" framework is acknowledged to be of use in conceptualizing complex systems, the focus of cognitive theory is primarily on cognitive factors in psychopathology and psychotherapy. Furthermore, cognitive concepts complement (and may even subsume) ideas such as "unconscious motivation" in psychoanalytic theory, and "reinforcement" or "conditioning" in behaviorism.

In the theory of cognitive therapy, the nature and function of information processing (i.e., the assignment of meaning) constitute the key to understanding maladaptive behavior and positive therapeutic processes. The cognitive theory of psychopathology specifically delineates the nature of concepts that, when activated in certain situations, are maladaptive or dysfunctional. Such idiosyncratic conceptualizations may be thought of as informal, personal theories. The cognitive conceptualization of psychotherapy provides strategies for correcting such concepts. Thus, the theoretical framework of cognitive therapy constitutes a "theory of theories"; it is a formal theory of the effects of personal (informal) theories or constructions of reality. In this respect, clinical cognitive theory overlaps to some extent with George Kelly's theory of personal constructs (Kelly, 1955).

Theory is essential to clinical practice. It has recently been reasoned that cognitive theory constitutes a unifying theory for psychotherapy and psychopathology (Alford & Norcross, 1991; Beck, 1991a). As we elaborate in Part II, we believe that the theoretical frameworks of effective psychotherapy must order the therapeutic components (treatments) and relevant psychological variables into a system of psychotherapy that constitutes a coherent model for general clinical practice. Unlike medical technologies, psychotherapeutic practices must be theoretically consistent if a therapist is to administer interventions in a manner that facilitates the patient's collaboration and empowerment. Such collaboration allows the therapist to enter the world of the patient, using the patient's own language and cultural context, while at the same time sharing the cognitive perspective. In this manner, cognitive therapy allows the person (through jointly developed homework assignments) to test cognitive theory in the context of his or her natural environment and belief structures.

Structure is necessary for collaboration. Patients must learn how improvement is obtained in order to view themselves as collaborative partners in the therapeutic enterprise. To teach their patients in this manner, therapists must themselves possess a theoretical rationale for specific treatment techniques. Otherwise, there is no structure on which to base the process of collaboration. Moreover, without theory the practice of psychotherapy becomes a purely technical exercise, devoid of any scientific basis. This issue is recognized by the most rigorous specialty boards that certify advanced competence in clinical practice. For example, the *Manual for Oral Examinations* of the American Board of Professional Psychology (ABPP) states explicitly that to earn the ABPP diploma, a psychologist must treat or make recommendations "in a meaningful and consistent manner, . . . backed by a coherent rationale" (ABPP, 1996, p. 3). (Although a "rationale" differs from a formal theory, it is hard to imagine how a coherent rationale can be developed apart from the empirically validated scientific theories of psychopathology and psychotherapy. This would certainly appear to be the case in standard clinical practice within the scientist/practitioner model.)

Cognitive therapy is the application of cognitive theory of psychopathology to the individual case. Cognitive theory relates the various psychiatric disorders to specific cognitive variables, and it includes a formal, comprehensive set of principles or axioms (delineated below). This chapter covers the following aspects of cognitive therapy and theory: (1) early development, (2) a formal statement of the theory, (3) theoretical directions and problems, and (4) future directions.

## EARLY DEVELOPMENT OF COGNITIVE THEORY

The historical origins of cognitive therapy, dating back to 1956, can be summarized as follows. Aaron Beck, in attempting to provide empirical support for certain psychodynamic formulations of depression (which Beck thought to be correct at the time), found some anomalies—phenomena inconsistent with the psychoanalytic model. Specifically, the psychoanalytic conceptualization (Freud, 1917/1950) asserts that depressed patients manifest retroflected hostility, expressed as "masochism" or a "need to suffer." Yet, in response to success experiences (graded task assignments in a laboratory setting), depressed patients appeared to improve rather than to resist such experiences (Beck, 1964; Loeb, Beck, & Diggory, 1971). This led Beck and his colleagues to further empirical studies and clinical observations, in an attempt to make sense of the anomalies. The eventual result was the reformulation of depression as a disorder characterized by a profound negative bias. The phenomenal content of this bias included expectations of negative outcomes (consequences of behavior) in the personal domain, and a negative view of self, context, and goals. Concurrently, attempts to modify the negative cognitive content and distortions were made, and these resulted in the development and evaluation of therapeutic strategies. Subsequently, the model was applied to other disorders to test the limits of the new formulation.

From this capsule summary, it can be seen that cognitive theory grew out of attempts to test specific theoretical tenets of psychoanalysis. When such evidence was not forthcoming, other explanations were considered. Thus, cognitive therapy from its inception was driven by theoretical interests. (See Arnkoff & Glass, 1992, for a more complete historical survey.)

## A FORMAL STATEMENT OF COGNITIVE THEORY

The cognitive theory of psychopathology and psychotherapy considers cognition the key to psychological disorders. "Cognition" is defined as that function that involves inferences about one's experiences and about the occurrence and control of future events. Cognitive theory suggests the importance of phenomenological perception of relationships among events; in clinical cognitive theory, cognition includes the process of identifying and predicting complex relations among events, so as to facilitate adaptation to changing environments. Previous statements developing and elaborating cognitive theory may be found in a number of publications (e.g., Beck, 1964, 1984b, 1987a, 1991b; Beck, Freeman, & Associates, 1990; D. A. Clark, 1995; Hollon & Beck, 1994; Leahy, 1995; Young, 1990).

The formal, comprehensive statement of cognitive theory presented here includes all assumptions that are both necessary and sufficient to the theoretical system, and forms the apex of the system (see Popper, 1959). Thus, all theoretical statements may be derived logically from the axioms (postulates or primitive propositions). No claim to truth is implied by the term "axiom." Rather, the reduction of a theory to axioms serves the important function of clarifying and defining a scientific theory. In the words of Popper (1959, p. 71),

> a severe test of a system presupposes that it is at that time sufficiently definite and final in form to make it impossible for new assumptions to be smuggled in. In other words, the system must be formulated sufficiently clearly and definitely to make every new assumption easily recognizable for what it is: a modification and therefore a *revision* of the system. (emphasis in original)

Popper (1959, pp. 71–72) suggests that few branches of science ever develop an elaborate, well-constructed theoretical system. He describes the requirements of such a rigorous system, which he terms an "axiomatized system," as follows: The axioms must be free from contradiction; they must be independent, so that axiomatic statements are not deducible from others within the system; the axioms must be sufficient to permit the deduction of all statements belonging to the theory; and, finally, the axioms must be necessary for derivation of the statements belonging to the theory. Consistent with these criteria, the formal axioms of cognitive theory are as follows:

1. The central pathway to psychological functioning or adaptation consists of the meaning-making structures of cognition, termed *schemas*. "Meaning" refers to the person's interpretation of a given context and of that context's relationship to the self.

2. The function of *meaning assignment* (at both automatic and deliberative levels) is to control the various psychological systems (e.g., behavioral, emotional, attentional, and memory). Thus, meaning activates strategies for adaptation.

3. The influences between cognitive systems and other systems are interactive.

4. Each category of meaning has implications that are

translated into specific patterns of emotion, attention, memory, and behavior. This is termed *cognitive content specificity*.

5. Although meanings are constructed by the person, rather than being preexisting components of reality, they are correct or incorrect in relation to a given context or goal. When *cognitive distortion* or *bias* occurs, meanings are dysfunctional or maladaptive (in terms of systems activation).[1] Cognitive distortions include errors in cognitive content (meaning), cognitive processing (meaning elaboration), or both.

6. Individuals are predisposed to specific faulty cognitive constructions (cognitive distortions). These predispositions to specific distortions are termed *cognitive vulnerabilities*. Specific cognitive vulnerabilities predispose persons to specific syndromes; cognitive specificity and cognitive vulnerability are interrelated.

7. Psychopathology results from maladaptive meanings constructed regarding the self, the environmental context (experience), and the future (goals), which together are termed the *cognitive triad*. Each clinical syndrome has characteristic maladaptive meanings associated with the components of the cognitive triad. All three components are interpreted negatively in depression. In anxiety, the self is seen as inadequate (because of deficient resources), the context is thought to be dangerous, and the future appears uncertain. In anger and paranoid disorders, the self is interpreted as mistreated or abused by others, and the world is seen as unfair and opposing one's interests. Cognitive content specificity is related in this manner to the cognitive triad.

8. There are two levels of meaning: (a) the objective or *public meaning* of an event, which may have few significant implications for an individual; and (b) the *personal or private meaning*. The personal meaning, unlike the public one, includes implications, significance, or generalizations drawn

---

[1]See Haaga and Beck (1995) for a review of the complexities and empirical status of the concept "cognitive distortion."

from the occurrence of the event (Beck, 1976, p. 48). The personal or private level of meaning was earlier presented as the concept "personal domain" (Beck, 1976, p. 56).[2]

9. There are three levels of cognition: (a) the preconscious, unintentional, *automatic* level ("automatic thoughts"); (b) the conscious level; and (c) the metacognitive level, which includes "realistic" or "rational" (adaptive) responses. These serve useful functions, but the conscious levels are of primary interest for clinical improvement in psychotherapy. (See the subsection "Three Cognitive Systems" in Chapter 3.)

10. Schemas evolved to facilitate adaptation of the person to the environment, and are in this sense *teleonomic* structures. Thus, a given psychological state (constituted by the activation of systems) is neither adaptive nor maladaptive in itself, but only in relation to or in the context of the larger social and physical environment in which the person resides.

These 10 axioms constitute the formal contemporary statement of cognitive theory. Several points of clarification may be useful. First, numerous specific hypotheses and/or models may be derived from the formal axioms (e.g., Beck, 1987a). Also, the axioms are interrelated, and may be combined to generate specific hypotheses. For example, cognitive content specificity (axiom 4) and cognitive vulnerability (axiom 6) have been combined to generate research hypotheses regarding the prediction of the onset of depression (Alford, Lester, Patel, Buchanan, & Giunta, 1995; Haaga, Dyck, & Ernst, 1991). A final point is that cognitive theory evolves (e.g., Beck, 1996); obviously, axioms are not intended as static principles. Rather, in the words of Popper (1959, p. 281): "Science never pursues the illusory aim of making its answers final. . . . Its advance is, rather, towards the infinite yet attainable aim of ever discovering new, deeper, and more gen-

---

[2]This level has been termed "implicational generic meaning" (Teasdale & Barnard, 1993, p. 217).

eral problems and of subjecting its ever tentative answers to ever renewed and ever more rigorous tests."

## THEORETICAL DIRECTIONS AND PROBLEMS

Several principles of cognitive theory included in the formal statements above are well known, such as the cognitive triad, cognitive content specificity, cognitive vulnerability, and the various "processing errors" or cognitive distortions. Other important aspects of the theory are less well known or are currently in the process of further development or refinement, and are therefore presented here. These include the nature of unconscious (automatic) processing of information; distal and proximal causes of fixation of attentional resources; and contemporary questions regarding the "constructivistic" nature of psychopathology. These are briefly reviewed in the subsections that follow.

### Automatic Cognitive Processing

The "cognitive revolution" in psychology has yielded numerous experimental findings (and concepts) that seem to parallel many clinically grounded observations of automatic cognitive processing. Also, the cognitive theory itself implicitly incorporates some of the relevant concepts, such as preattentive processing, cognitive capacity, and "unconscious" processing. For example, contemporary cognitive psychologists have used the term "cognitive unconscious" to describe mental structures and processes that operate outside phenomenal awareness, yet determine conscious experience, thought, and action (Kihlstrom, 1987, p. 1445; Meichenbaum & Gilmore, 1984).

There is no theoretical reason that the cognitive processes relevant to psychopathology must operate entirely within conscious phenomenal awareness. Consider the following sequence: situation to belief to interpretation to affect to behavior (see Figure 1.1). To elaborate, existing belief structures or schemas are activated by environmental circumstances. Schematic (meaning) processing, whether conscious or unconscious, generates an interpretation. The specific interpretation leads to affect, which is followed by specific behavior, which in turn modifies the original situation.

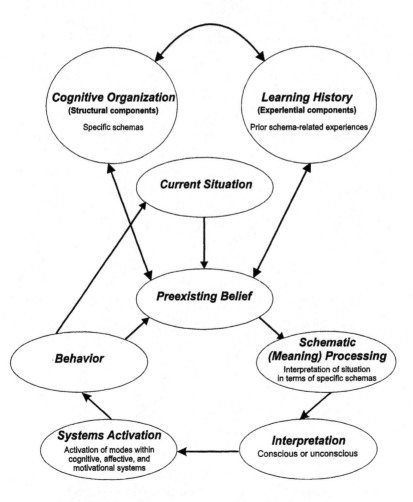

FIGURE 1.1. Schematic processing of information.

The concepts "automatic thoughts" and "cognitive unconscious" possess many common features. Though clinical observation has found that automatic thoughts are often rather easily admitted into conscious awareness (Beck, 1976; Beck, Rush, Shaw, & Emery, 1979), the theoretical status of the notion of "automaticity" suggests that such cognitive processing is perhaps best labeled "preconscious." Since conscious awareness is a logical prerequisite to conscious control (see Kihlstrom, 1987, p. 1448), cognitive therapists naturally employ clinical techniques designed to make (initially) largely unconscious automatic thoughts (e.g., faulty attributions) more subject to conscious awareness through cognitive techniques, such as distraction or redirection of the attentional resources (see Beck et al., 1979). This approach avoids direct attempts to "control" thoughts, since such attempts often result in effects opposite to the ones intended (see Wegner, 1994).

Though the empirical status of nonconscious processing in psychopathology is at present inconclusive, several lines of research have supported the presence of automatic biased processing in the anxiety disorders (Foa, Ilai, McCarthy, Shoyer, & Murdock, 1993; Logan, Larkin, & Whittal, 1992; MacLeod, 1991; MacLeod & Mathews, 1991; McNally, 1990), as well as in depression (Mineka & Sutton, 1992). Also, a recent controlled study of memory bias for catastrophic associations (e.g., "dizzy"–"faint") in panic disorder found biased memory in both conscious (explicit) and nonconscious (implicit) memory processes (Cloitre, Shear, Cancienne, & Zeitlin, 1992).

## Transfixed Attentional Resources

One of the unresolved problems in basic cognitive experimental research is how to account for the fixation of attentional resources, particularly in the anxiety disorders. Beck (1985a) has theorized generally that a functional impairment in the normal activity of cognitive organization occurs in panic disorder and probably in other disorders as well (e.g., depression and bipolar disorder), and that this impairment leads to reduction in the ability to focus attention properly or concentrate (p. 1433).

Two other factors may also help explain how attentional resources become fixed in panic disorder. First, the presence of unconscious cognitive processing as discussed above may explain this in part. To the extent to which cognitive content exists at a level inaccessible to conscious awareness, it would appear that correction of distortions would not be possible (Kihlstrom, 1987). The fixation of attentional processes to threat stimuli, and the elaborative and interpretative processes to threat themes, are accounted for in terms of automaticity; such processes are automatic in the sense of being unconscious. (It should be noted that McNally, 1995, has articulated three different meanings of the term "automatic" in the context of the anxiety disorders. Automatic processes may be "capacity-free," meaning that they proceed effortlessly and without interference with concurrent processes; they may be "unconscious," or outside awareness; and/ or they may be "involuntary," meaning outside conscious control. McNally concludes that automatic processes in the anxiety disorders are never capacity-free, are sometimes unconscious, and are always involuntary.) However, the fact that such processes are unconscious does not mean that they cannot be modified in therapy. The treatment of unconscious processes in cognitive therapy has been described previously: "The patient begins to recognize at an experiential level that he has misconstrued the situation. . . . this mechanism is perhaps analogous to what the psychoanalysts call making the unconscious conscious" (Beck, 1987b, p. 162).

Second, it has been suggested that there exists an innate and generally adaptive tendency to establish and widen "orientation," or the range of phenomena to which an organism attends (see Kreitler & Kreitler, 1982, 1990). To the extent to which this is true, it would seem adaptive that such an orientation process could be deactivated by catastrophic meanings, since it is genetically adaptive to focus all available attentional resources on threats to immediate survival. However, during this process the innate and generally adaptive tendency to widen orientation (i.e., to construct and entertain other meanings) would be foreclosed. Consistent with cognitive theory, the person suffering from anxiety becomes "stuck" in a mode crucial for survival in situations of actual threat, and the ability to entertain other interpretations is thus blocked (Beck, Emery, & Greenberg, 1985).

## The Constructivistic Nature of Meaning

An issue of the *Journal of Consulting and Clinical Psychology* was devoted largely to "constructivist" psychotherapeutic approaches (Mahoney, 1993). In that series of articles, leading cognitive theorists addressed the importance of constructivist approaches to psychotherapy and psychopathology. For example, Ellis (1993) contrasted earlier rational–emotive theory with more recent formulations, which he described as "distinctly constructivist and humanistic" (p. 199); and Meichenbaum (1993) suggested that constructivism is "a third metaphor that is guiding the present development of cognitive-behavioral therapies" (p. 203).

Meichenbaum (1993) has defined the constructivist perspective as "the idea that humans actively construct their personal realities and create their own representational models of the world" (p. 203). Similarly, Neimeyer (1993) states that the core of constructivist theory is "a view of human beings as active agents who, individually and collectively, co-construct the meaning of their experiential world" (p. 222). Consistent with this, Beck et al. (1979) wrote: "Perception and experiencing in general are *active* processes that involve both inspective and introspective data" (p. 8; emphasis in original). The meaning a person attaches to a situation, or the way an event is structured (or constructed) by a person, theoretically determines how that person will feel and behave (see Beck, 1985a). Moreover, cognitive theory not only suggests the "construction" of reality; it also postulates cognitive content specificity, in which specific emotional responses (normal and abnormal) are associated with different *kinds* of constructions (Beck, 1976, 1985a).

Put simply, normal human behavior is theorized to be dependent upon a person's ability to apprehend the nature of the social and physical environment within which the individual is situated. Cognitive therapy is often misunderstood as taking only a "realist" perspective. However, the cognitive perspective posits at the same time the dual existence of an objective reality and a personal, subjective, phenomenological reality. In this manner, the cognitive view is consistent with contemporary conditioning theories, which postulate both external physical stimulus characteristics and cognitive mediations of these (Davey, 1992).

An important point has been articulated by Mahoney (1989, p. 188), who has expressed concern over dichotomizing "constructivistic" theory: "People do, indeed, co-create their realities, just as their realities co-create them. The future of heuristic theories in psychology must, however, liberate itself from the pendular swings of that dualism and somehow embrace the complexity of our position as both subjects and objects of construction." Mahoney differentiates between "critical constructivists," who do not deny the existence of a real world, and "radical constructivists," who are idealists (in the philosophical sense of the term) and argue that there is no reality beyond personal experience.

In social contexts where phenomenological realities intersect, there are multiple personal realities as well as an objective physical reality or context within which the subjective realities reside. These "realities" are equally real, in the sense that they are part of what exists. Quite obviously, this topic raises the issue of the nature of human consciousness and metacognition.

When a person experiences stress or a psychological disorder, information relevant to the prepotent schemas will be abstracted selectively, and the person will base his or her interpretation of the entire situation on this selective abstraction (see Dalgleish & Watts, 1990; Logan et al., 1992; MacLeod & Mathews, 1991). In addition, given the same input of data, the psychopathological state will shape the interpretations much more systematically than will the nonpsychopathological state.

A person with a psychological disorder is in a purely constructivist state. However, in the more normal state, a person is both a constructivist and an empiricist/realist. Thus, when a person is reacting normally, the instantaneous reaction/cognition to, say, a chest pain may be schema-driven ("I am having a heart attack"); however, on quick reflection (metacognition), the person discards this hypothesis. The cognitive therapist, when it comes to therapy with a patient, oscillates between two states:

1. Understanding empathy involves a constructivist state.
2. As a realist/empiricist, the therapist gets the patient to focus more on what is going on (thus freeing the patient from the dominance of the dysfunctional schemas), to search for more information, and to generate alternative explanations for a particular event.

## FUTURE DIRECTIONS

### Personality Theory (and Modes)

#### Defining Personality

An important future direction for cognitive theory is in the further development of personality theory. Personality is perhaps the most complex and idiographic of the cognitive constructs. Consistent with a view of personality as complex biological behavior, Ross (1987, p. 7) has suggested the following comprehensive definition: "a composite construct that stands for the sum total of people's actions, thought processes, emotional reactions, and motivational needs, through which they, as genetically programmed biological organisms, interact with their environment, influencing it and being influenced by it." Thus, "personality" is the term we apply to specific patterns of social, motivational, and cognitive–affective processes, the individual study of which constitutes the various specialized areas of psychological research.

In addition to providing a definition of personality that is consistent (at least in principle) with basic psychological science, the formulation above articulates a somewhat novel view of what elements must be included in a contemporary scientific conceptualization of personality as a unifying or organizing construct for complex human behavior. A comprehensive theory would include the various systems of complex human behavior, such as behavioral, cognitive, motivational, and emotional systems, and these must be related to biological and social environments. Such a theory would have to describe how the component systems interrelate and influence one another, how they have evolved to adapt to the environment, and how the mechanisms of stability and change operate. Ross (1987, pp. 33–34) argues that although there are "minitheories" concerning, respectively, anxiety, learning, motivation, memory, interpersonal behavior, emotion, and other systems, no theorist has yet developed a comprehensive theory of personality. Below, we describe a salient step toward developing such a comprehensive theory.

## A Cognitive Theory of Personality

Beck et al. (1990) have suggested that cognitive, affective, and motivational processes are determined by the idiosyncratic structures, or schemas, that constitute the basic elements of personality. The schemas are said to be operative normally, as well as in both Axis I and Axis II disorders. Except for mental retardation, the Axis II disorders are the personality disorders, which include the antisocial, avoidant, borderline, dependent, histrionic, narcissistic, obsessive–compulsive, paranoid, schizoid, schizotypal, and "not otherwise specified" varieties (American Psychiatric Association, 1994). The schemas typical of the personality disorders are theorized to operate on a more continuous basis than is typical in the clinical syndromes. This notion may provide an integrating concept that has heretofore been lacking in theories of personality and personality disorder.

Regarding the central role of the schema construct in the cognitive theory of personality disorders, it is interesting to note that several theorists (e.g., Horowitz, 1991; Kazdin, 1984) have similarly observed that concepts of cognitive psychology encompass or explain the operation of numerous systems (affect, perception, behavior), and thus may serve to provide a common language to facilitate the integration of certain psychotherapeutic approaches (as asserted in Alford & Norcross, 1991, and Beck, 1991a). Furthermore, personality itself may be thought of as an integrating concept. The task of identifying an efficacious language to explain the interrelationships among various systems is analogous in the present context to the problem of integrating the various effective systems of psychotherapy. Given this, the observation that cognitive concepts are involved in both areas of integration is not surprising.

The schema concept has been adapted as a structure around which to organize and understand the operation of the various psychological systems, and it appears to suggest a commonality in the ethological function of these systems. When personality disorders are viewed as chronic idiosyncratic patterns of systems based on the activation of maladaptive schema, schematic or meaning processing is theorized to control the operation of psychological systems.

The cognitive definition of personality includes individual schematic processes, which theoretically determine the operation of the major systems of psychological analysis (e.g., motivation, cognition, emotion, etc.). The cognitive perspective would emphasize characteristic patterns of a person's development, differentiation, and adaptation to social and biological environments. These patterns are composed of relatively stable organizations of schemas, which account for the stability of cognitive, affective, and behavioral systems across time and situations. These specialized schema systems are conceptualized as the basic components of personality. Specific suborganizations of these basic systems are termed *modes* (Beck, 1996). Modes provide the content of the mind, which is reflected in the constructions or perspectives. The modes consist of the schemas that contain the specific memories, the algorithms for solving the specific problems, and the specific representations in images and language that form the perspectives. Disorders of personality are conceptualized simply as hypervalent maladaptive systems operations (coordinated as modes) that are specific to primitive strategies. The operation of dysfunctional modes, though presently maladaptive, presumably served in more primitive contexts to secure adaptation/survival. The various modes activate programmed strategies for carrying out basic categories of survival skills, such as defense from predators, the attack and defeat of enemies, procreation, and energy conservation (Barkow, Cosmides, & Tooby, 1992; Baron-Cohen, 1995, Ch. 2).

This perspective may appear at first to be an obvious approach, until one compares it to that which has been commonly advanced. Both cognitive and noncognitive (e.g., Skinnerian) psychological theorists have applied the Darwinian principles of genetic survival to include evolutions of complex behavior or cognitive systems. The earlier (radical) behavioral writings of Skinner made explicit analogies between the selection of a species' characteristics and the selection of an individual's behavior by its consequences. Similarly, Beck et al. (1990) have theorized that the evolution of the structural (schematic) organization of the specific traditional personality modes (avoidant, antisocial, dependent, etc.) was grounded in ethological principles.

In accord with Ross (1987), this view of personality is necessarily conceptually incomplete, as is the basic science of the respective psychological systems or domains of analysis. However, advances in understanding personality disorders will parallel the advances in understanding those aspects of schematic processing in memory, comprehension, and attention/perception (as examples) that may vary from person to person, and that may constitute vulnerability to personality disorder (see MacLeod & Mathews, 1991). A domain-specific conscious or unconscious schematic activity, such as interpersonal interaction, emotion, or cognition, has been selected (by evolutionary processes) to facilitate specific types of processing. The type of processing selected is the one most likely to be adaptive under the environmental conditions that activated that particular mode.

The operation of a mode (e.g., anger, attack) across diverse psychological systems (emotion, motivation) is determined by the idiosyncratic schematic processing derived from an individual's genetic programming and internalized cultural/social beliefs. To take an example from perception, studies have shown that olfaction involves several neuronal systems, including nasal receptor cell spatial patterns of activity, the olfactory cortex, and the entorhinal cortex (which combines signals from other sensory systems). The inclusion of other sensory systems results in a perception that has a unique meaning, since the perceived scent is associated with memories specific to a given person (Freeman, 1991). Personality is similarly idiosyncratic and based on systems activation at "higher" cortical levels. Consistent with this point, Flanagan (1992, p. 222) notes that the personality (or self)

> is the joint production of the organism and the complex social world in which she lives her life. Presumably, it would be idle labor to look for type-identical neural maps of the self-representations of different individuals. This is not because self-representation is not neurally-realized. It is because the phenomenological particularity of self-represented identity suggests neural particularity.

Put differently, although the self cannot exist apart from neurons, the uniqueness of the self as experienced suggests that distinctive neural patterns constitute the personality of each individual. Moreover, personality cannot in any case be understood by "reducing" it to the physiological level (i.e., patterns of neurons), since the intrinsic meaning of such neural patterns can only be discovered within personal phenomenological experience.

In summary, cognitive theory considers personality to be grounded in the coordinated operation of complex systems that have been selected or adapted to insure biological survival. The various systems manifest continuity across time and situations, and have been described in psychological writings as the numerous personality "traits" and "disorders." More abstractly, these consistent coordinated acts are controlled by genetically and environmentally determined processes or structures, termed "schemas." The schemas are essentially both conscious and unconscious "meaning structures"; they serve survival functions. To be effective, schematic processing must be adaptive to immediate social and environmental demands through adaptive systems coordination and operations. When environmental circumstances change too rapidly (as from pre- to postindustrialization, or from hunting to agricultural societies), previously adaptive strategies continue to operate, so that a poor fit may develop. For example, traits suited for the aggressive hunting of wild game may not fit a social environment that values the patient cultivation of agricultural products. Much of what we refer to as "personality disorder" probably has its origins in the evolution of strategies for survival that are relatively less effective, or actually maladaptive, in present environments (Beck et al., 1990, Ch. 2; Gilbert, 1989). Further articulation of the nature of personality is an important future direction for cognitive theory (see also Pretzer & Beck, 1996).

## The Evolving Nature of Cognitive Theory

The specific components of cognitive theory employed in therapy with a given patient are specific to the goals or aims of the therapist, given the contextual situation (i.e., the patient's characteristics, such as personality and affective responsivity). Thus, cognitive theory regarding strategies for treatment of a particular case depends on the goals of the cognitive therapist, as derived from the individual case conceptualization.

In its general form, cognitive theory stipulates that symptomatic improvement in psychological disorder results from modification of dysfunctional thinking, and that durable improvement (relapse reduction) results from modification of maladaptive beliefs. Within this broad definition of cognitive therapy, the application of selected theoretical formulations supported by basic cognitive experimental research would be considered cognitive psychotherapy. Thus, the cognitive therapist, in modifying patient thinking and beliefs, is free to borrow theoretical concepts from basic cognitive experimental research without violating the fundamental principles of cognitive therapy. In this manner, cognitive theory evolves along with basic research on the nature of cognition.

# CHAPTER TWO

# Metatheory

Certain misconceptions about cognitive therapy on the part of psychotherapy integrationists (and others) have contributed to the failure to appreciate the integrative nature of cognitive theory and therapy (see Gluhoski, 1994). In a review of a major edited volume on psychotherapy integration, A. A. Lazarus (1995b) noted the following: "It seemed to me that specific orientations were often inaccurately presented and unfairly judged, that caricatures of certain approaches were presented, that straw men (or is it persons?) were set up and demolished" (p. 401). Therefore, this chapter and Chapter 3 clarify other specific metatheoretical and theoretical aspects of cognitive therapy.

Much of philosophy has historically addressed poorly defined questions. Yet the right question is as important as the right answer. Indeed, without the correct question or a meaningful question, one cannot arrive at a sensible answer. Many questions and misconceptions about cognitive therapy seem to miss the mark by addressing the subject in a much too simplistic, reductionistic, or dichotomous (either–or) manner. For example, it is obviously simplistic to ask, "Does an airplane fly because it has wings, or because it goes fast?" However, it may not seem so simplistic to ask, "Does a person experience panic because of cognitive factors, or because of physiological ones?" Yet the two questions are equally inadequate.

In addition to such dichotomizing, a number of other, interrelated issues, regarding the philosophical foundations of cognitive therapy should be clarified. These include (1) the nature of theory; (2) types of "causes"; (3) the nature of cognition; (4) cognition as a clinical–theoretical bridge; and (5) cognition and the therapeutic relationship. These specific issues are discussed in the sections that follow.

## THE NATURE OF THEORY

As a cognitive phenomenon in itself, the nature of theory is of particular interest to us. In this section, we briefly discuss six common misconceptions about the nature of theory. These include (1) the false dichotomy between clinical and scientific theory; (2) the false dichotomy between theories of simple and of complex phenomena; (3) the fallacy that metaphors or analogies (e.g., the computer as human cognition) are the equivalent of scientific theories; (4) the necessarily diverse, intrinsically limited, and often contradictory nature of the metaphors or analogies used to describe a natural phenomenon; (5) circularity in basic psychological terms; and (6) subjectivity in psychological science.

Regarding the first misconception, cognitive therapy has been characterized as a "clinical" rather than a "scientific" theory (Teasdale & Barnard, 1993, p. 211). However, in the context of clinical phenomena, experimental psychopathologists observe the same phenomena as clinical practitioners (see Stein & Young, 1992). Indeed, to the extent to which this is not the case, the observation of the nonclinical theorists may lack ecological validity. Therefore, separate criteria do not appear tenable in the evaluation or categorization of clinical versus scientific theory. Rather, criteria such as parsimony, scope of applicability, empirical validity, testability, and internal consistency apply to theories in general. Moreover, since clinical cognitive theory is an axiomatized system, the distinction between clinical and scientific theories cannot accurately suggest different degrees of precision or testability. As described by Popper (1959) (and demonstrated in detail in Chapter 1 of this volume), a theory is clarified and defined through its reduction to a number of specific axiomatic statements.

The second point concerns the false dichotomy between theories of simple and of complex phenomena. As orderly presentations of perceptual experience, scientific theories are systematic descriptions of the world—quantitative or qualitative statements of experience (see Popper, 1959, p. 94). In most cases, greater or lesser degrees of precision (prediction) are possible, depending on the level of complexity (number of controlling variables) of the phenomena that are the subjects of scientific analyses.

Thus, in studying humans (and particularly in studying complex aspects of humans such as cognition), the degree of complexity involved is greater than, for example, that involved in studying the swing of a pendulum. In the latter case, relationships between time and the pendulum's motion can be described quantitatively. In the former case, precision of the type obtained in describing the pendulum's movement is not possible. This is particularly true in the exceptionally complex science of cognitive content specificity and cognitive processes in psychopathology. Nevertheless, the theories of each respective phenomenon are equally "scientific," according to the typical understanding of the term (Popper, 1959). The fact that certain domains of scientific analysis are complex, and others relatively simple, does not logically confer a different scientific status on one or the other. This point is analogous to the first point above regarding the false distinction between clinical and scientific theory.

Our third point concerns the distinction between metaphors or analogies and theories. Basic scientists often attempt to simplify complex domains of scientific analysis by using analogies or metaphors as explanatory devices. This is generally a quite reasonable practice. However, the uncritical use of such devices can have important disadvantages. For example, in a recent review of a new book in cognitive science, Sternberg (1993) noted that cognitive scientists seem to have little to say about how people actually think in their everyday lives. Furthermore, he attributed this absence of ecological validity to a remarkable error in thinking on the part of cognitive scientists themselves: There often appears to be a confusion between the use of computer metaphors to explain human cognitive processes, and human processes as such. In Sternberg's words, "What started off as a metaphor (the machine) for an object of study (the human) perhaps will one day replace the object of study" (1993, p. 1274).

The human mind uses computers to serve only as information management tools. Computational analogies may never lead to an understanding of how the mind works, since the brain is not a digital computer (Searle, 1990). Indeed, computers as extensions or creations of the mind (tools of the mind) may shed no more light on mental processes than, say, eating utensils enlighten us about nutrition. Utensils assist us in manipulating food, and computers in calculating. However, calculations are possible without computers, and nourishment may be obtained without the aid of utensils. Indeed, one might even use one tool analogy (e.g., the spoon) in place of the other (the computer) to account for cognition, and still retain about as much explanatory power! Consider this example: "The mind scoops up information like a spoon." Compare it with the following: ". . . schematic models are used to *compute* propositional meanings [IMPLIC–PROP] which can, in turn, be sent back [PROP–IMPLIC] to *feed* further model-based processing. In many important respects this cycle is the *central engine* of human cognition" (Teasdale & Barnard, 1993, p. 76; emphasis added). In the first analogy, the mind is like a "scoop." In the second, it "computes," "feeds," and becomes an "engine."

The extent to which such analogies assist us in understanding the actual content or mechanisms of the mind is as yet unclear. However, Searle (1990) has provided logical reasons to suggest that such analogies are "ill defined" (p. 35). His argument is not that they are wrong, but rather that they lack a clear sense. To summarize (in part) his line of reasoning, because computational analogies are at much too high a level of abstraction, they fail to capture the concrete reality of intrinsic intentionality and consciousness. As examples, Searle (1990) suggests that the "information" in the brain or mind is always specific to some modality, such as thought, vision, hearing, or touch.

In operating a computer, the human operator encodes information in a manner that he or she, as the *outside agent*, then interprets both syntactically and semantically. As Searle (1990, p. 34) notes, "the hardware has no intrinsic syntax or semantics: It is all in the eye of the beholder." It is just this fundamental difference between computational theories and clinical cognitive theory that explains the failure of computational theories to adequately incorporate intrinsic states of consciousness into their basic theoretical axioms (if such axioms are set forth at all). Thus, cognitive content specificity (to take one axiomatic example) cannot be reduced to any aspect or fact that can be meaningfully compared to a digital computer.

Fourth, continuing with the topic of metaphors as scientific hypotheses or models, Pepper (1963, p. 269) has differentiated the "world hypothesis" from other hypotheses: "Other hypotheses are implicitly, if not explicitly, limited to a local problem in hand or, as in the special sciences, to a special field of subject matter." Within a given domain of scientific interest, scientific conceptualizations are not typically consistent with a single root metaphor or analogy (see Oppenheimer, 1956). To take an example previously noted elsewhere (Alford, 1993b), the physical science conceptualizations of light utilize "particle" and "wave" metaphors simultaneously. Similarly, complex psychological phenomena (such as human cognition) do not behave in ways that allow for simple, unitary metaphorical categories. Thus, although a number of metaphors may be found useful to make the formal statement of cognitive theory concrete, neither cognitive theory nor its object of study may be limited to any single analogy.

Our fifth comment on the nature of theory concerns basic theoretical terms. The term "schema," as one such basic term in cognitive theory, is used to explain and predict individual differences in the functioning of complex psychological systems (e.g., perception, motivation, affect, and cognition). Thus, we may refer generally to schemas as "basic structures that integrate and attach meaning to events," and we may also state that schemas "mediate strategies for adaptation."

To analogize, the basic term "reinforcement" serves in behavioral theories to explain how (rather than "that") human behavior is modified during an organism's adaptation to complex environments. The radical behavioral theoretical account of changes in response probability is in terms of contingencies of "reinforcement." "Reinforcement" is then defined as changes in response probability, so that a somewhat circular explanation is offered. Thus, the term "reinforcement" is a basic or undefined term.

Perhaps the alternative to circular theory is linear theory. Which is better may depend on the nature of the phenomenon (or phenomena) being described. If the phenomenon is linearly related to other phenomena, then the linear explanation is preferable; if it is related to other phenomena in a reciprocally determined, feedback–feedforward manner, then the circular theory is appropriate. Thus, given the "biopsychosocial" nature of psychological phenomena, R. S. Lazarus (1991b, p. 30) is probably correct that circularity is inevitable in psychology. Relatedly, it is important to avoid confusing precision with the use of inappropriately reductionistic definitions. Terms must be applied at a level of analysis commensurate with the phenomena under study.

The issue of circularity is related to that of undefined terms. To define a phenomena is to demarcate its boundaries, to specify its location in space, or to identify its conceptual characteristics. A central point of this volume is that cognitive theory is integrative in nature. Cognitive therapy subsumes a broad scope of phenomena and includes observations from many vantage points. This characteristic of cognitive theory requires a level of analysis that includes the entire range of variables implicated in the generation of meaning. Thus, the concept "meaning" is properly understood as itself a consequence of various systems; it is caused by multiple variables that themselves are in need of explanation. The level of analysis of cognitive theory is a legitimate (useful) level, in that lawful relationships have been identified at this higher level of complexity.

As Laing (1967, pp. 29–33) has noted, "theories can be seen in terms of the emphasis they put on *experience*, and in terms of their ability to articulate the relationship between experience and behavior" (emphasis in original). In cognitive therapy, variables within the external environment and internal phenomenological experience are integrated into a unified, coherent theory for clinical practice. This position has been articulated both in early formulations (e.g., Beck, 1964) and in more recent ones (Beck, 1991b). For example, in explaining the proximal origins of the cognitive construct "automatic thoughts," Beck (1991b, p. 370) implicates both internal and external variables: "The relevant *beliefs* interact with the symbolic *situation* to produce the automatic thoughts" (emphasis in original). Thus, the fundamental philosophical position of cognitive therapy, and the basic theoretical constructs consistent with its philosophical position, integrate internal (phenomenological) and external (environmental) dimensions.

The final issue concerns the place of "subjectivity" in psychological science. In science, objectivity is defined in terms of agreements among the subjective perspectives (observations) of individual scientists. Thus, objectivity is derived from subjectivity, and in this sense is subordinate to it. Consistent with the primacy of cognition, certain terms and causal variables in cognitive theory refer to private (subjective) phenomena (Alford, Richards, & Hanych, 1995). These include interpretative processes and experiences of the individual person. For example, schemas are defined as meaning-assignment structures of cognition, and the term "meaning" is then defined as the person's interpretation of a given context and the relationship of that context to self. Some may object to these clinical theoretical terms and definitions by alleging that they lack "specificity," or that they suggest an intrinsic "unscientific" subjectivity.

Goldman (1993, p. 368) has explicated this issue as follows:

> Not all words in the language (perhaps very few) can have "reductive" definitions. There must be exits from the circle of purely verbal definitions. . . . It should not be surprising that the meanings of some words, especially those addressed here, should be attached largely to subjective experience rather than behavioral criteria. Why shouldn't words like "conscious," "aware," and "feeling" be associated in common understanding with subjectively identifiable conditions rather than behavioral events (cf. Jacobson, 1985a, 1985b)?

Extending this line of reasoning, Searle (1993) has argued that it is possible to have an epistemically objective science of consciousness, even though the domain of consciousness is ontologically subjective. He views consciousness as entirely caused by brain processes, and emphasizes that consciousness is not some extra substance or entity. Rather, consciousness is a higher-level *feature* of the whole system (Searle, 1992; 1993, p. 312). Consistent with this view, the axioms of cognitive theory presented earlier describe the nature (and interactions) of different levels, aspects, and functions of human consciousness (or mind) in a clinical context (see Searle, 1993).

## CAUSES

The term "cause" has several meanings in philosophy and psychology (see White, 1990). As reviewed by White (1990), the notion of "efficient cause" refers to prior events' or external compulsion's bringing about an effect. Early scientific explanations generally focused on efficient causation, as scientists explained how external variables compelled subsequent things to happen. Such explanations were reductionistic or atomistic in their metaphysical assumptions (White, 1990). In psychological theorizing, such assumptions are questionable and certainly inadequate to the entire subject matter. The phenomena in which the experimental psychopathologist is interested are at a level of complexity or interrelatedness that generally does not lend itself to efficient causal analyses.

Final causal analyses focus on the consequences or end products of the phenomena to be explained, as well as on the manner in which such consequences of the phenomena may play a causal role in its appearance. Final causes have been emphasized in behavioral theory, in that *reinforcement* is said to be the end result or "purpose" for which an act occurs (cf. White, 1990, p. 4). Rachlin (1992) suggests that final causal analyses are necessarily or intrinsically less precise than are efficient causal analyses. This is the case because final causal analyses must explain the history of the development of a particular psychological phenomenon; therefore, environmental contexts and variables from the past must be considered (Rachlin, 1992, pp. 1378–1379). For example, in cognitive theory, the efficient causal explanation for the maintenance of a depressive episode would include the negative bias in cognitive organization that influences the processing of incoming information. The precise manner in which the negative cognitive bias has evolved over time, and the circumstances that selected this particular cognitive programming, may never be entirely explained, although evolutionary processes presumably selected such mechanisms in the same manner as other adaptive mechanisms are selected. Thus, the cognitive theory of psychopathology and psychotherapy includes both efficient and final causal explanations; as such, it encompasses multiple levels of causal analysis.

Behaviorists such as Dougher (1993) have spoken of the need to identify external causes of behavior, and have suggested that cognitive mechanisms "are in need of explanation and cannot be used as explanations in their own right" (p. 204). Although we would agree that final causal analyses are desirable, and that "the analysis (of behavior) remains incomplete" (Dougher, 1993, p. 204) unless external and/or distal causes are articulated, scientific analyses of complex open systems always remain incomplete. It is obvious that a *complete* analysis would require the inclusion of the "Big Bang" plus all prior and subsequent events (Alford, Richards, & Hanych, 1995).

Another source of complexity faced by cognitive theorists is the causal status of an individual's intentions, goals, and the meanings that are attached to events. Radical behavioral theorists have argued that one's personal thoughts and feelings are "inevitable reactions to the world rather than as causes of actions" (Dougher, 1993, p. 205). However, cognitive theory sees the person as a potential "free agent" or "independent variable." Although causes of the free action can often be identified, a person may become cognizant of the causes of a given behavior that may be inconsistent with specific goals; the person may then choose to change that behavior to make it consistent with specific goals (values). The activation of the metacognitive system, defined as the sum total of all variables of which a person is aware, may acquire causal status in itself (Alford, Richards, & Hanych, 1995).

The task faced by cognitive theorists is to devise an adequate cognitive theory to account for the origins of psychopathology, and, relatedly, to account for the clinical correction of such disorders. To do so in a comprehensive manner requires an understanding of the operation of human psychological functioning from diverse levels of analysis, including perspectives from various related scientific disciplines (e.g., brain and evolutionary biology, sociology, genetics, and basic social–cognitive psychology).

To tie together so many diverging scientific fields will require an interdisciplinary or "systems" approach commensurate with the complexities of actual clinical practice. A comprehensive theory would eventually include relationships among the various systems of complex human behavior, such as the behavioral, cognitive, "motivational," and emotional systems; these must be related to biological and social systems. The theoretical concept of "mode," presented in Chapter 1, elaborates such relationships (Beck, 1996). Such a theory would describe how the component systems interrelate and influence one another, how they have evolved to adapt to the environment, and how the mechanisms of stability and change operate. Cognition provides an integrating framework for such a systems (contextual or relational) theory.

## THE NATURE OF COGNITION

Cognitive theory is descriptive of a broad range of clinical phenomena (variables) observed in actual clinical practice. The context of actual clinical practice is a rather complex environment that includes interacting systems at many levels, particularly interpersonal/social variables (see Beck, 1988b; Beck et al., 1979, Ch. 3). The purpose of cognitive theory is to provide conceptual tools for effective action or practice in such clinical contexts. It also explicates the factors or processes responsible for the development, maintenance, correction, and prevention of psychopathology.

Cognitive theory explicates the role of *cognition* in the interrelationships among clinically relevant variables, such as emotion, behavior, and interpersonal relationships. Cognition as currently defined includes all theoretical structures necessary to support the processing of information. Yet it is more than that, since cognition may include "thinking about thinking" (metacognition), along with the objects or events that constitute the content of thinking. As such, cognition is clearly a contextual, interactional construct (cf. Werner, Reitboeck, & Eckhorn, 1993). It coordinates systems and is transactional.

To say that cognition is "contextual" simply means that its processing and phenomenological content is determined by or responds to activating circumstances within the environment. At the same time, a person's conscious phenomenal experience (perception) can take on an emergent causal status. Thus, it is equally reasonable to ask, "What causes consciousness?" and "What does consciousness *cause*?"

The human organism can act with intention and purpose to modify its environment or its own response to this environment. Thus, the philosophical stance of cognitive theory on the issue of "free will" recognizes cognition as a mechanism that can in part be determined or controlled by external variables. Yet, at the same time, the nature of human consciousness includes the potential for causality and creativity. Indeed, without this potential, there would be no new scientific theories from which to derive testable hypotheses for empirical scientific research!

Cognitive theory does not suggest that the cognitive apparatus is capable of directly grasping (or "representing") reality. Internal and external phenomena impinging upon a human nervous system interact with that system. Thus, human conscious experience does not unilaterally construct the world (as radical social constructionists may suggest); rather, it consists of an interaction *with* the world or environment. Even scholarly critics of cognitive theory would agree on this most basic point. For example, Coyne (1994) has accurately noted the importance of analyzing not only "what is in the head," but also "how the head is in transaction with the interpersonal world" (p. 403).

English and English define a cognitive schema as "the complex pattern, inferred as having been imprinted in the organismic structure by experience, that *combines with the properties of the presented stimulus object or the presented idea* to determine how the object or idea is to be perceived or conceptualized" (quoted in Beck, 1964, p. 562; emphasis added by us). As elaborated in "The Nature of Theory" above, the analogy to information-processing systems (computers), though perhaps of some heuristic value, falls short in many respects. Computers do not directly enter into transactions with the world in the same manner as human cognition does. Rather, data are managed entirely in terms of the aims of the programmer(s).

Put differently, cognition mediates between the environment and the human organism. Presumably, through natural selection it evolved to do so. In actively *adapting to* the world, the human cognitive system engages in transactions with the natural environment, whereas "computer behavior" is determined by variables over which computers experience no direct control. Thus, cognitive theory incorporates ecological as well as information-processing principles or characteristics.

Consistent with the position above, Searle (1994) has recently suggested that even to argue that computational metaphors for the mind are false is to concede too much! He makes this case on the basis of the failure of theorists who employ computational metaphors to distinguish between phenomena that are intrinsic and ones that are observer-relative. Regarding this matter, he concludes: "So the question, 'Is consciousness a computer program?' lacks a clear sense. . . . Computation exists only relative to some agent or observer who imposes a computational interpretation on some phenomenon. This is an obvious point. I should have seen it 10 years ago, but I didn't" (Searle, 1994, p. 103). The identical point is made by Goldman (1993): "Our ordinary understanding of awareness or consciousness seems to reside in features that conscious states have in themselves, not in relations they bear to other states" (p. 367).

## COGNITION AS A CLINICAL-THEORETICAL BRIDGE

In conducting general clinical treatment of a psychological disorder, the psychotherapist relies primarily on verbal communication to facilitate correction of the disorder. This is the case whether the psychotherapist takes a behavioral, a psychodynamic, or any other established psychotherapeutic approach. Thus, one commonality among the various psychotherapies is that therapy involves communication, or the exchange of information, between therapist and patient.

This exchange of information constitutes a cognitive process between the participants. The information exchange typically includes the following: (1) emotional states, (2) behavioral symptoms, (3) expectations for improvement, and (4) experiences and meanings attached to experiences. Furthermore, the clinical exchange of information (communication) occurs on both implicit (nonconscious) and explicit (conscious) levels of awareness on the part of both the client and the therapist. Cognitive theory as a "theory of theories"—a theory that articulates the manner in which personal theories (cognitive schemas) determine the operation of other psychological systems (Beck, 1996; Kelly, 1955)—stipulates that alterations in cognitive processes determine the impact of therapy.

Even when clinical therapeutic interaction includes the application of other nominal therapies (such as behavioral techniques or the free association of conscious cognitive products), psychotherapy is indisputably an exercise of information exchange. The exchange between therapist and patient can focus on operant conditioning concepts. Therapist and client can discuss likely positive or negative consequences of actions, and during the therapy session itself they may construe such consequences within the client–therapist context. They may also consider psychoanalytic concepts, such as sexual and aggressive impulses and the manner in which such impulses are recognized (and adaptively directed) in the client's life. Or they may discuss humanist notions of self-actualization. However, regardless of content, the process of therapy commonly referred to as the "therapeutic relationship" or "alliance" is in essence simply an exchange of information between therapist and client—nothing more (or less).

Cognitive primacy, a basic metatheoretical position of cognitive therapy, is consistent with one fundamental observation: that all other psychological processes are explained by means of cognitive concepts. This point appears so obvious that perhaps its implications are commonly overlooked. For example, "experiential" therapists convey their therapeutic approach primarily by means of verbal (cognitive) constructs, not experiential ones. Whether as psychological scientists or as a nonscientists, humans cannot convey or *organize* processes such as "behavior," "experience," "emotion," or "the therapeutic relationship" except through cognitive constructs. No other psychological function provides this particular organizing function. Thus, there is an obvious parallel between (1) the cognitive formulations or theoretical organizations of diverse psychological processes (cognition, affect, behavior) by behavioral scientists, and (2) the psychological organizations of humans in their natural environments who may be the subject of study and theorizing by the behavioral scientists. In either case, cognition alone provides meaning (or coherence) to the various other basic psychological processes. This central issue is developed further in Chapter 3.

## COGNITION AND THE "THERAPEUTIC RELATIONSHIP"

Given the problems of definition and specificity associated with the concept "therapeutic relationship," this topic might easily be considered as a philosophical, rather than a theoretical, issue. For this reason, it is included in the present chapter. In cognitive therapy, as in any verbal (vs. pharmacological) approach to psychological treatment, a social or interpersonal environment exists within the therapy session (Beck et al., 1979, Ch. 3; Safran, 1984). The term "therapeutic relationship" or "alliance" simply refers to this interpersonal environment. (It might be noted, however, that the term "therapeutic" in the commonly used reference to the "therapeutic relationship"—as a "common factor" across psychotherapies [e.g., Castonguay & Goldfried, 1994, p. 164]—*assumes* that the relationship will have a positive interpersonal impact. The question "Is the therapeutic relationship therapeutic?" is tautological; it is equivalent to the question "Is effective treatment effective?")

Arkowitz and Hannah (1989, p. 149) note that time-limited dynamic therapy (TLDP) regards the therapeutic relationship as a necessary prerequisite to *and* the major vehicle for change. What does it mean to say this? Arkowitz and Hannah (1989, p. 149), citing Strupp and Binder (1984), state that "the meaning and function of any technical intervention is determined by the context of the therapeutic relationship." In cognitive therapy, the therapist obviously addresses those maladaptive styles (cognitive, affective, behavioral) that a patient manifests during treatment sessions (i.e., in the therapeutic relationship). The patient–therapist relationship, however, does not constitute the whole context of patients' lives. Arkowitz and Hannah state:

> As these authors [Strupp & Binder] emphasize, the learning that takes place is relationship-based rather than cognitively based. In TLDP, as troublesome patterns become activated

within the context of the patient–therapist relationship, the patient can explore and correct the erroneous assumptions underlying his or her maladaptive behavior. (p. 149)

Yet it would be more accurate to say that the learning that takes place is *both* relationship-based and cognitively based. These are simply different levels of abstraction. The term "relationship-based" refers to the person of the therapist along with the patient. The term "cognitively based" refers to the patient's learning. These two levels are interactive; how can there be learning that is not cognitive?

Presumably, the changes that take place within the patient–therapist relationship will generalize to other relationships. However, discrimination may occur. A patient may learn or display a set of interaction patterns within the patient–therapist relationship that are specific to that particular relationship. On the surface, it would appear preferable to utilize therapeutic strategies that are designed to produce generalization to contexts outside the patient–therapist relationship. As Frank (1980, p. 336) has pointed out,

regularities between therapist interventions and patient responses within an interview can have little practical relevance. Evaluation of therapeutic outcome, whether from the standpoint of the patient, the patient's social unit, or society, depends solely on changes in the patient's behavior and subjective state outside the therapeutic interview.

Another concern about the patient–therapist relationship relates to the issue of the collaborative stance. When the therapeutic relationship is seen as *the* major vehicle for change, the therapist takes on a larger role than when the patient–therapist relationship is viewed as just one of many important relationships in the patient's life. Put differently, there is no necessary reason for problems in the patient–therapist relationship to be relevant to those that may arise between the patient and other significant persons in his or her life. Of course, this is precisely the assumption underlying psychodynamic approaches: Problems in relating to others will be manifested in relating to the therapist and can then be corrected within the patient–therapist relationship.

However, problems in the patient–therapist relationship are not *necessarily* relevant to those arising in other contexts. The special demand characteristics and expectancies within the therapeutic context are clearly different from those within a patient's natural environment. Monica Harris (1994) has provided a comprehensive review of many such factors in an important article, which begins with the following observation:

> The therapeutic relationship is unlike any other. In the hope of seeking relief from life's problems, one person divulges passions, pains, and bitter memories to an almost total stranger. The relationship is nonreciprocal and temporary and *does not follow the traditional norms that govern our other interactions with people.* (p. 145; emphasis added)

It might be more useful to view the patient–therapist relationship in the same way as one would view a student–teacher relationship in, say, learning to play the piano. One might say that the student–teacher relationship is the major vehicle for improvement, and (with a talented student) even for becoming a great pianist. The reactions of the capable teacher to the various performances of the student pianist could be viewed as analogous to a therapist's reactions to a patient's interpersonal performance. Yet, in either case, it would appear incorrect and perhaps even aggrandizing for the therapist/teacher to attribute improvement solely to the relationship between therapist/teacher and client/student. To do so seems to negate the influences of other contexts, such as those encountered during homework exercises, as well as the characteristics of the client/student. Consistent with the humanist tradition, cognitive theory places much of the responsibility for change on the individual who seeks treatment from the cognitive therapist.

Despite these considerations, the cognitive therapist does not minimize the importance of interpersonal relationship factors between therapist and patient. Indeed, these factors are given considerable attention in cognitive therapy, and have been reviewed elsewhere (as necessary but not sufficient). For example, Beck et al. (1979) provide a detailed review of the therapeutic relationship, including the following components: (1) therapist characteristics (warmth, accurate empathy, genuineness); (2) the therapeutic interaction (basic trust, importance of rapport); (3) the therapeutic collaboration (eliciting "raw data," authenticating introspective data, investigating underlying assumptions, etc.); and (4) "transference" and "countertransference" reactions (Beck et al., 1979, Ch. 3, pp. 45–60). Interested readers may also want to consult Wright and Davis (1994) for a review of relationship factors in cognitive therapy.

## CONCLUSIONS

The metatheoretical positions of cognitive therapy are neither simplistic nor reductionistic. Cognitive metatheory (1) resolves a number of false dichotomies concerning the nature of theory; (2) provides a complex and multifaceted view of the meaning of "causes" in psychopathology; and (3) acknowledges the importance of multiple categories of causal variables (e.g., social, environmental, cognitive) that are implicated in psychopathology and are necessary to the implementation of effective psychotherapy. Cognition provides a theoretical bridge to link the contemporary behavioral, psychodynamic, humanistic, and biopsychosocial perspectives of psychopathology and effective psychotherapy. Finally, a cognitive theoretical view of the therapeutic relationship—a "common factor" in effective psychotherapy—has been presented.

# CHAPTER THREE

# Cognitive Mediation of Consequences

There is much overlap between cognitive theory and behavior therapy (Beck, 1970a). For example, in regard to the importance of consequences of behavior, cognitive theory is not inconsistent with radical behavioral theory. Indeed, Skinner (1981) presented cogent arguments and evidence that behavior is often selected by its consequences. As elaborated more fully in Chapter 6, cognitive theory holds the potential to integrate principles of both operant conditioning and classical conditioning into a more unified theory of behavior change (see also Bouton, 1994).

This chapter focuses on one aspect of learning that relates to a cognitive conceptualization—that is, conflicts between short-term and long-term consequences in psychopathology. (We often refer to these below as "temporal-consequences conflicts," for the sake of brevity.) The chapter addresses the important theoretical question of resolving the "neurotic paradox," described below. Our analysis integrates basic behavioral conceptualizations (and data from experimental learning studies) into cognitive theory, and may prove valuable in further broadening the scope of cognitive clinical theory and practice. We theorize that the metacognitive level—an intrinsically subjective state of consciousness—potentially mediates conflicts between short-term (immediate) and long-term (delayed) consequences.

## TEMPORAL CONFLICTS OF CONSEQUENCES

An interesting theoretical puzzle that exists within learning theory may be explicated by cognitive theory. The puzzle was first suggested in an article by Mowrer and Ullman (1945), reviewed in detail below. The question evolved and was refined in articles by Renner (1964) and Ainslie (1975), and clinical implications were suggested by Shybut (1968). These articles considered the question of how organisms master the environmental complexities that result from temporal changes or irregularities in the relationship between behavior and its consequences.

An increase in explanatory power was apparent from 1945 to 1975 (in the above-cited articles). For example, Shybut (1968) suggested clinical implications of temporal-consequences conflicts and related impulsivity, and Ainslie (1975) provided an early cognitive formulation for the resolution of such conflicts that included attentional and conceptual routes to private control (pp. 479–480). However, little has since been written by clinical cognitive theorists on the question of how such learning takes place.

In discussing the lack of attention to earlier behavioral formulations, Eifert, Forsyth, and Schauss (1993, p. 109) have observed that in paradigm shifts (parallel to the shift from behavioral to cognitive theory) in other sciences, "accuracy and achievements of earlier theories are maintained and further developed in the new theory." Indeed, the further integration of basic behavioral conceptualizations (and data from experimental learning studies) into cognitive theory may prove valuable in further broadening the scope of cognitive clinical theory and practice. This is the intent of the analysis that follows.

## Relationships between Behavior and Outcome

The behaviorist Donald Whaley (1978) identified four logical relationships between behavior and its long-range outcomes: (1) persevering when one should, (2) persevering
when one should not, (3) quitting when one should, and (4)
quitting when one should not. Whaley added that although
the long-term outcomes are not always readily apparent, they
do nevertheless exist, and therefore there may be "right" and
"wrong" actions in terms of positive or negative consequences
(see cognitive theory axioms 5 and 10, Chapter 1). Thus,
Whaley was a realist in this regard. Since effective environmental conditions are not always present to guide behavior,
it is not always evident whether it would be better to persist
in specific activities that may not be immediately rewarding.
It may be that one fails to persist when persistence would be
rewarded. Conversely, Whaley theorized that one often per-
sists when one should not, thereby wasting valuable resources, getting no positive outcome, and perhaps even being
punished for the efforts. In terms of cognitive theory, one
often assigns meaning to context in a manner that does not
properly control the behavioral system (see axioms 1 and 2,
Chapter 1). This dysfunction typically occurs at the automatic
level, with little conscious participation (see axiom 9).

The nature and function of human consciousness appear
to be largely ignored within contemporary theories of behavior therapy. For example, the term "consciousness" does not
appear in the subject index of the 753-page edited volume
*Theories of Behavior Therapy*, published by the American Psychological Association (O'Donohue & Krasner, 1995). (The clos-
est entry is "consciousness raising," a topic found in a chapter
on feminist theory.) Conditioning models generally focus on
an observer's view of relationships among events; neither the
individual's perception of behavior–reinforcement relationships, nor their qualitative content or *meaning*, are addressed

by noncognitive behavioral theory (e.g., Brewer, 1974; S. C. Hayes & Wilson, 1993; Moore, 1984; Skinner, 1969, 1981).

For the radical behaviorist or noncognitive conditioning theorist, behavior is entirely a function of past associations. This results in relatively poor explanatory power in accounting for the resolution of temporal-consequences conflicts. By contrast, cognitive theory advances principles of human conscious experience as explanatory constructs (e.g., Beck, 1976). In delineating some features of human consciousness, Searle (1993) observes that one important aspect is "unity": Consciousness appears as one unified experience. He suggests this aspect of consciousness is identical to that described by Kant as "the transcendental unity of apperception," and to what contemporary neurobiology calls "the binding problem" (Searle, 1993). Important in the present context is that the unity of consciousness implies an intrinsic temporal element. That is, "the organization of our consciousness *extends over more than simple instants*. So, for example, if I begin speaking a sentence, I have to maintain in some sense at least an iconic memory of the beginning of the sentence so that I know what I am saying by the time I get to the end of the sentence" (Searle, 1993, p. 314; emphasis added). We return to consider this issue in the subsection "Three Cognitive Systems," following a review of the role of temporal-consequences conflicts in psychopathology.

## Empirical Studies of Temporal Conflicts of Consequences

The observation that the *immediate* consequences of behavior, as opposed to the *delayed* consequences, exert relatively more influence on the probability of the occurrence of future similar responses has been made both in the experimental learning laboratory and in clinical situations.[1] Indeed,

[1]Portions of this historical review are adapted from Alford (1984).

Kimble (1961) cited numerous animal studies and five independent lines of evidence showing that "responses spatially or temporally near reinforcement are learned more quickly than responses remote from reinforcement" (p. 140). Likewise, laboratory studies of human behavior have shown that when reward is effectively delayed, learning is slower than when reward is not delayed (Salzman, 1951).

Similar conclusions are found within cognitive formulations. For example, Bolles (1972) described the "law of prior expectancy," and suggested that organisms generate predictive relationships between behavior and consequences. He suggested that these prior expectancies impose constraints on adaptive learning, particularly when reinforcement events (positive outcomes or consequences) are delayed in the presence of responses or cues that signal such consequences (Bolles, 1972, p. 405). Moreover, studies confirm that dimensions of behavior other than rate of learning are subject to this temporal effect, including faster running speed following acquisition trials in rats given immediate (vs. delayed) reinforcement (e.g., Calef, Haupt, & Choban, 1994).

In discussing the role of the timing of consequences in clinical behavior problems, Goldfried and Davison (1976, p. 26) mention "the so-called neurotic paradox"; this refers to behaviors' having immediate positive consequences but long-term negative ones, as in the case of alcoholism or drug addiction. The person who receives immediate reward for behavior that has negative long-term consequences may develop a "behavior problem," because immediate consequences are often more powerful in shaping behavior. Likewise, if a person fails to obtain an immediate reward for engaging in an activity that has significant long-term positive consequences, then that behavior will perhaps fail to persist in the person's behavioral repertoire (Malott, 1980). This conflict between short-term and long-term consequences is theoretically implicated not only in alcoholism and drug addiction, but in obesity, impulse control disorders, and numerous other psychopathological conditions.

As Renner (1964) pointed out, Mowrer and Ullman (1945, p. 87) were the first to demonstrate experimentally that the timing of consequences is related to "non-integrative behavior," or "behavior which has (long term) consequences which are usually more punishing than rewarding." The subjects in Mowrer and Ullman's experiment were 21 laboratory black rats, placed on a restricted diet to reduce their body weight by 15%. They were first trained to run to food at the sound of a buzzer. Next, a "rule" was made that the subjects were not to touch the food for a period of 3 seconds following its appearance in the trough. Touching the food within this 3-second period of time resulted in a 2-second shock from the floor of the training apparatus. The 21 rats were then randomly divided into three equal groups as follows: a 3-second group, a 6-second group, and a 12-second group. These three groups were treated in exactly the same manner except for how soon the shock was administered following violation of the 3-second rule. One group was punished (shocked) immediately after touching the food within the 3-second time period; a second group was punished 3 seconds after touching the food during the taboo period; and a third group was punished 9 seconds after the transgression. Possible responses were labeled "normal," waiting 3 seconds before eating; "neurotic," avoiding the shock by not eating at all; and "delinquent," eating within the 3-second period and getting shocked.

Results showed that as latency to negative consequences increased, normal responses decreased. In other words, "the capacity of the rat to compare and balance the good and bad consequences of an act is very dependent upon the temporal order and timing of these consequences" (Mowrer & Ullman, 1945, p. 76). These authors concluded that "if an immediate consequence is slightly rewarding, it may outweigh a greater but more remote punishing consequence. And equally, if an immediate consequence is slightly punishing, it may outweigh a greater but more remote rewarding consequence" (p. 87).

Ainslie (1975), in noting the conceptual importance of this early study in understanding behavior disorders, stated that "the growing number of behavior therapists who deal with impulsiveness rarely mention this model or specifically attribute impulsiveness to the discounting of delayed reward" (p. 469). Studies by Mischel (1961, 1974) and Shybut (1968) were among the few to test the theory that psychological disorders are associated with conflict between short- and long-term consequences. These studies have clearly shown greater psychological adjustment in persons who have favorably resolved this conflict, in that their behavior is directed to more desirable long-term consequences rather than less desirable (smaller) short-term consequences; those who maximized reinforcement over time showed greater adjustment. Subjects were asked to choose among actual alternatives in realistic situations. Those preferring larger delayed rewards were shown to score higher on measures of social responsibility, resistance to temptation, personal adjustment, intelligence, and achievement orientation (Mischel, 1961, 1974).

In a study using patients whose diagnoses included a wide range of psychological and psychiatric problems, Shybut (1968) compared 30 normal individuals with 45 severely disturbed inpatients in a Veterans Administration hospital setting. The tendency to delay gratification was measured by allowing subjects to choose between immediate smaller reinforcement and larger reinforcement to be given after a period of time. Results showed that the three groups differed significantly in terms of choosing the long-term but larger consequences. The more severely disordered subjects were more readily attracted to the immediate but less desirable reinforcement (Shybut, 1968).

These studies support the view that conflict between short-term and long-term consequences of behavior may lead to clinical disorders. Mischel (1974, p. 288) suggests that in the achievement of long-range goals and psychological adjustment, behavior and outcome must be mediated in some way, since immediate reinforcement for goal-directed behavior may not always be present.

## Empirical Studies of Mediation

A study by Ayllon and Azrin (1964) directly addressed this issue of the complementary roles of instructions (rules) and reinforcement. In this study, the "mediator"—verbal instruction—was external to the patients, who were attempting to develop adaptive behavior. Two experiments were conducted. In the first, participants were 18 psychiatric inpatients who consistently failed to pick up their eating utensils at mealtimes. Following a baseline period of 10 meals, reinforcement in the form of candy, cigarettes, and extra coffee or milk was given to patients who picked up all utensils. After 20 consecutive meals, instructions were added in which attendants told the patients to pick up the utensils in order to obtain the reinforcement. Results showed that little improvement was obtained with the operant consequences alone, but that when instructions were added along with the reinforcement, a significant improvement was noted. Twenty inpatients similar to those in the first experiment participated in the second experiment. No instructions and no consequences were arranged during the first 10 meals. During the next 110 meals, instructions were given, but no consequences. During the next 110 meals, operant consequences were added along with the instructions. Results showed that patients receiving instructions alone increased responding for a short time, but then declined. This short-term improvement was attributed to their previous learning history of reinforcement for following instructions. When operant consequences were added along with instructions, between 90% and 100% of patients made the appropriate response, and this percentage persisted throughout the remainder of the time this procedure was maintained.

The study described above was conducted by investigators within a radical behavioral (rather than a cognitive) paradigm, and they targeted overt verbalizations. Of course, the *processes* of change were not directly measured, and similar studies were subsequently conducted according to a cognitive conceptualization. For example, positive clinical effects have been obtained when self-instructional training procedures have been used with a wide range of clinical problems, particularly in children (Kendall, 1977, 1993; Kendall & Braswell, 1985; Kendall & Finch, 1976).

Self-instructional training generally aims to modify covert verbalization or "self-talk." A typical example of this procedure is found in a study of a 9-year-old impulsive boy (Kendall & Finch, 1976). In the first step of treatment, the therapist modeled performance of tasks and talked aloud to himself, with the patient observing. Self-instructions involved step-by-step verbalizations about the problem definition, problem approach, focusing attention, and coping statements. Then the patient performed the task, talking aloud to himself in the manner in which he had observed the therapist talking. For example, in the task of adhering to topics of conversation, the patient said,

> "What should I remember? I'm to finish talking about what I start to talk about. O.K. I should think before I talk and remember not to switch. If I complete what I'm talking about before I start another topic I get to keep my dimes. I can look at this card (cue) to remind me." (Kendall & Finch, 1976, p. 854)

Next, the therapist performed an additional task while whispering to himself. Finally, the patient performed the task with instructions to talk to himself. Target behaviors were untimely switches, or shifts, from one task behavior to another before the former behavior was complete. Improvement was noted in all target behaviors at posttreatment and at a 6-month follow-up.

Similarly, Meichenbaum and Cameron (1973) found that when schizophrenics were trained in gradually more complex self-instructional responses, improvement was obtained on a variety of indices, including "sick talk," abstract thinking, digit recall, and perceptual integration. Mahoney and Mahoney (1976) found covert assertive statements about weight control to be an essential component of their comprehensive treatment program to develop self-control in obese clients. And Novaco (1975) found that the use of self-statements significantly added to the therapeutic efficacy of a treatment program for controlling anger and "hostility."

To take other examples of studies testing the effects of cognitive (verbal) mediation, O'Leary (1968) found that "cheating" could be reduced through the use of self-instructions. The experimenter in this study told participants that they would get one marble each time a figure (a blue circle, a yellow circle, a blue triangle, or a yellow triangle) appeared on a screen *and* they pressed a key. They were also told that they would get one of three prizes, depending on the number of marbles they collected, with better prizes being given for a greater number of marbles. After learning this, participants were told that they should press the key only if specific figures appeared. Those who were taught to say out loud, "Yes, it should be pressed" (when the specific figure appeared) or "No, it shouldn't be pressed" (when the specific figure did not appear) cheated significantly less than children in the control condition did.

Monahan and O'Leary (1971) observed that the self-instructions in the O'Leary (1968) study were effective in controlling a behavior that led to immediate positive consequences, but that also would lead to, or might lead to, future aversive consequences. In a successful replication of O'Leary's study, Monahan and O'Leary (1971) investigated possible differential effects of self-instructions emitted 1 second versus 9 seconds before the opportunity to cheat. No differences that could be attributed to temporal delay were found, and the effects of self-instructions generalized to other forms of rule-breaking behavior not specifically targeted in the experiment. In a related study, Mischel and Patterson (1976) designed a distractor called "Mr. Clown Box" to tempt children away from assigned tasks. They found that resistance to temptation could be enhanced by having children verbalize instructions such as "No, I'm not going to look at Mr. Clown Box" and "I want to play with the fun toys and Mr. Clown Box later."

The effective treatments employed in studies such as those described above were based on the premise that the alteration of "verbal behavior" can result in the alteration of behavioral disorders. Such treatments may result in mediation between the long- and short-term consequences of maladaptive behavior patterns. Meichenbaum (1976) used the neurological concept "final common pathway" in an analogy to describe the general mechanism of behavior change operating in these studies; he stated that this common pathway is the "alteration in the internal dialogues in which our clients engage" (p. 224). In so doing, he suggested a departure from previous behavioral accounts, in that the internal dialogue is a cognitive formulation. Next, we consider one example in which this paradigm shift (from behavioral theory to cognitive theory) is most apparent.

## Verbal versus Cognitive Mediation

There are differences as well as similarities between behavior therapy and cognitive therapy. One fundamental difference is seen in the manner in which cognitive versus behavioral therapies deal with intrinsically private phenomena, such as delusional beliefs (Alford & Beck, 1994). Put simply, behaviorists limit treatment to the modification of "verbal behavior" (e.g., Ayllon & Haughton, 1964; Liberman, Teigen, Patterson, & Baker, 1973; Wincze, Leitenberg, & Agras, 1972), whereas cognitivists focus on the goal of belief modification (e.g., Alford, 1986; Chadwick & Lowe, 1990; Hole, Rush, & Beck, 1979). A brief review of findings in this area will serve to highlight this difference.

Stahl and Leitenberg (1976) raised the following question relevant to these two perspectives: "It has been clearly demonstrated [by behaviorists] that delusional speech can be controlled through operant techniques. An unresolved question is whether delusional 'thought' is modified by the same methods" (p. 234). Marzillier and Birchwood (1981) suggested that delusional thinking and beliefs are not necessarily modified by therapies that focus on topographical verbal behavior, and they distinguished between delusional "verbal behavior" and delusional beliefs. Himadi, Osteen, Kaiser, and Daniel (1991) utilized a changing-criterion design, and found that cognitive (belief) changes do not necessarily occur during the application of noncognitive behavioral approaches for the modification of delusional verbalizations. In this study, conviction of delusional beliefs was assessed in a single-subject design. Ten questions that reliably elicited delusional material were developed; statements used in conviction ratings corresponded with the structured interview questions used in eliciting delusional verbalizations. Thus, delusions targeted for verbal modification were the same as those for which conviction of delusional belief was assessed. Though a stepwise decline in the frequency of delusional responses (verbalizations) was found, no changes were obtained on measures of the subject's conviction ratings of delusional beliefs.

These findings have important theoretical as well as clinical implications (Alford & Beck, 1994). The Himadi et al. (1991) study experimentally addressed the question of whether there are concomitant changes in conviction of delusional belief when delusional verbal behavior is targeted and successfully eliminated. These studies (Himadi, Osteen, & Crawford, 1993; Himadi et al., 1991) found that behavioral treatment of verbalizations does not insure the reduction in delusional beliefs as such. Thus, the presence of delusional ideation is not synonymous with delusional verbalizations. Follow-up studies have replicated the initial results (Himadi et al., 1993).

Differences in theoretical level of analysis have for some time differentiated the traditional behavioral and cognitive approaches to psychopathology and psychotherapy. Verbal behavior is still the sole target of noncognitive behavior therapists (see L. J. Hayes & Chase, 1991), rather than a focus on the cognitive content (specific beliefs) and cognitive processes (cognitive distortions) that give rise to such behavior. In the words of radical behaviorist Jay Moore (1984, p. 3), "any contribution of a private phenomenon is presumably linked at some point to a prior public event that has endowed the private phenomenon with its functional significance." As another example, clinical behavioral theorists S. C. Hayes and Wilson (1993, p. 287) write: "Neither meaning nor understanding is a mental event, and the ground of verbal communication between the two is not an idea of the mind."

Behaviorists limit their focus to the "objective" realm, while giving relatively little or no attention to the phenomenological perspective of the individual patient. By contrast, the cognitive clinical theorist takes the position that the more important focus of analysis is the level of personal or private meaning. Again, the two levels of meaning posited by cognitive theory (see axiom 8, Chapter 1) are (1) the objective or public meaning of an event, which may have few significant implications for an individual; and (2) the personal or private meaning. The personal meaning, unlike the public meaning, includes the significance or generalizations drawn from the occurrence of events. The notion of "verbal behavior" represents only the public level, but (according to cognitive theory) the personal or private meaning level is necessary for an understanding of psychopathology and effective psychotherapy. This approach places the cognitivist more within the sphere of common-sense analyses shared by the patient who seeks psychotherapy (cf. Goldman, 1993).

The discussion above shows that cognitive theory is clearly distinguishable from the behavioral theories, which do not address phenomenal consciousness or personal meaning. With great clarity, Brewer (1974) identified the essential feature that distinguishes conditioning theory from cognitive theory. Conditioning theory refers to the idea that learning occurs in an automatic, unconscious fashion. In contrast, cognitive theory explains conditioning in terms of conscious awareness of the relationship between the conditioned stimulus (CS) and the unconditioned stimulus (UCS) (classical conditioning), or the reinforcement contingency (operant conditioning) (see Brewer, 1974, p. 2).

To return to the issue of temporal consequences, within noncognitive behavioral theory there is no way (apart from environmental modification) to account for the resolution of conflicts between short-term and long-term consequences. Behavioristic perspectives give no theoretical attention to phenomenological perceptions (e.g., assignment of personal meaning); no construct in behavioral theory explains the function of cognitive biases or distortions (e.g., incorrect perception of response–reinforcement relationships). In the clinical behavioral treatment of disorders, temporal-consequences conflicts can only be resolved by modification of the environment, so as to insure that adaptive responses are immediately reinforced and maladaptive responses are punished (or extinguished).

## HOW COGNITION MEDIATES CONSEQUENCES

Having described studies consistent with a link between temporal-consequences conflicts and psychological disorders, we now return to the axioms of cognitive theory. These principles explicate numerous relationships and provide theoretical explanations for the resolution of such conflicts. Briefly, by means of cognitive schemas, the human organism assigns meaning to events and processes information that is antecedent to strategies for adaptation. The central pathway to psychological adaptation is to be found in this meaning-making function of cognition. It is important in the present context to note that "meaning" includes the constructed relationship between a behavior (emitted within a given context) and the instrumentality of that behavior in reaching a person's goals.

Cognition is implicated in controlling or directing behavior so as to maximize positive consequences (both short-term and long-term), and it provides a theoretical account of behavior–reinforcement relationships and associative relationships that is consistent with contemporary research (see Bouton, 1994; Powers, 1992). Although meanings are constructed by the person rather than being direct components of reality, they are relatively accurate or inaccurate in relation to a given context and a person's goals. This corresponds to external aspects of radical behavioral formulations, such as Whaley's (1978) four possibilities: persisting when one should (correct), persisting when one should not (incorrect), quitting when one should (correct), and quitting when one should not (incorrect). When individuals engage in faulty cognitive constructions (cognitive distortions), the resulting behaviors may lead to long-term negative outcomes.

As outlined above, the history of psychological theorizing suggests an evolution from (1) conditioning to (2) "verbal-mediational" to (3) cognitive theories to explain the mediation of temporal-consequences conflicts. The active role of the organism is an intrinsic part of both cognitive theory and Skinner's notion of the operant; however, the level of analysis of cognitive theory includes both external (contextual) and phenomenological dimensions. Regarding "classical conditioning," Bouton (1994) has recently reviewed how context provides meaning for Pavlovian cues by the reduction of ambiguity. This leads to more differentiated, adaptive responding. Memories of previous trials of cued responding in diverse contexts guide the differentiated responding. Bouton's findings support cognitive theory in that, when behaviors change, responses are not "unlearned"; rather, they are under the control of higher cortical processes (such as memories of context) rather than of stimulus–response (S-R), reflexive processes (see Bouton, 1994). Thus, information processing is antecedent to strategies for adaptive responding.

## Three Cognitive Systems

As described above, cognitive theory is a theory about the role of cognition in the development, maintenance, treatment, and prevention of clinical disorders. Cognition includes the entire range of variables implicated in the processing of information and meaning. In the present context, "meaning" refers to consciousness of relationships between behavior and consequences.

In axiom 9 (Chapter 1), cognitive theory stipulates three cognitive systems (or levels): (1) the preconscious, unintentional, *automatic* level; (2) the conscious level; and (3) the metacognitive level. Although the notion of "distancing" has been a central concept within cognitive clinical theory for some time (e.g., Beck, 1976, pp. 242–245), the relationship between this clinical construct and basic cognitive science has not previously been explicated. Distancing is an active, regulatory process that involves the activation of the metacognitive level of functioning. Flavell (1984) has defined the term "metacognitive" as pertaining to any knowledge or cognitive activity that takes as its object, or regulates, any aspect of any cognitive enterprise. Similarly, Sternberg (1994) identifies "metacomponents" as one of three kinds of information-processing components of memory-analytic abilities. He defines them as higher-order thought processes involved in planning what one is going to do, monitoring it while one is doing it, and evaluating it after it is done. . . . Examples of metacomponents are recognizing that one has a problem in the first place, defining what the problem is, setting up a strategy to solve that problem, monitoring one's strategy as one is seeking to implement it, and evaluating the success of the strategy after one has completed implementing it. (p. 221)

Interestingly, each of these steps is explicitly included in the clinical practice of cognitive therapy. For example, the standard protocol for cognitive therapy of depression includes identifying negative attitudes, pinpointing the most urgent and accessible problem, developing homework strategies, monitoring (recording) homework strategies between therapy sessions, and reviewing problems and accomplishments since the preceding session (Beck et al., 1979, pp. 409–411).

In cognitive theory, the metacognitive level (1) selects, (2) evaluates, and (3) monitors the further development of schemas for particular situations, tasks, or problems. It is the cognitive level that regulates the lower cognitive levels. Thus, in addition to the automatic (or preconscious) level, cognitive theory posits the conscious level wherein a person can report cognitive content. Furthermore, the metacognitive level allows the person in cognitive therapy to report processing operations/errors (e.g., arbitrary inference, personalization) as well as cognitive content.

Multiple levels of functioning have likewise been suggested by neobehavioral learning theorists (e.g., Amsel, 1989). In discussing this issue, Amsel (1989) suggests that there appear to be at least two levels, which have been given the following different names: "non-cognitive versus cognitive; S-R versus cognitive; procedural versus declarative; procedural versus propositional (semantic and episodic); habit systems versus memory systems" (p. 84). In a critique of these models, he argues that they do not lead to the consideration or examination of transitions between levels, nor to recognition of the possibility of simultaneous operation of both levels.

However, cognitive theory has been influenced by Freud's concept of the hierarchical structuring of cognition into primary and secondary processes. In this manner, cognitive theory bridges the gap between the two levels of analysis. That is, cognitive theory incorporates both the unconscious level of functioning, which has been the primary focus of conditioning, and also the "higher" levels (the conscious and metacognitive levels), which have been of particular interest to most cognitivists.

This concurrent focus on both levels of analysis can perhaps be attributed to the observation that cognitive theory originated in a context of pragmatic exigencies associated with clinical practice. In this context, primary (automatic thought) as well as secondary (rational response) levels were found useful in understanding and treating clinical disorders. Thus, both S-R, unconscious, or habit systems (automatic cognitive processing) and conscious (rational response) levels are included in cognitive theory (Alford, 1993b; Alford & Carr, 1992; Moretti & Shaw, 1989).

## Clinical Cognitive Theory and Basic Research

Cognitive therapists consider not only clinical observation, but basic cognitive experimental research, as relevant to clinical theory (e.g., Beck, 1991a; Segal, 1988; Stein & Young, 1992). For example, recent basic experimental work by Epstein (1994) elucidates the cognitive clinical perspective on the cognitive systems. Epstein makes the following distinctions between the experiential system (ES) and the rational system (RS): The ES is based on associationistic connections and the RS on cause-and-effect connections; the ES engages in more rapid processing and is oriented toward immediate action (associated with short-term consequences), and the RS is characterized by slower processing and more delayed action (associated with long-term consequences); the ES is experienced passively and preconsciously, and the RS actively and consciously. In short, the RS is a conscious, more discriminating, analytic mode, and it can correct the more primitive mode (ES) (S. Epstein, personal communication, October 12, 1994). The resolution of conflicts between short-term and long-term consequences may be accounted for theoretically by the coordination of these cognitive systems.

The formulation above is consistent with and provides empirical support for clinical cognitive theory (Epstein, Lipson, Holstein, & Huh, 1992). As presented previously, there are three levels of information processing within the cognitive system: the automatic, the conscious, and the metacognitive levels. (Note that the distinction between the conscious and the metacognitive levels is made in terms of active vs. passive monitoring of conscious experience. The term "metacognitive" is used to convey the active, deliberative control function of conscious awareness.) The automatic level corresponds roughly to the ES, and the metacognitive level to the RS. The metacognitive level involves "thinking about thinking" and is of most relevance in the present context, since it is the level responsible for learning about and attending to delayed consequences.

In clinical cognitive theory, metacognition results from the operation of the *conscious control system*, a system that has evolved to override primal thinking, affect, and motivation. This system is responsible for setting and attaining long-term goals, as well as for problem solving. Moreover, the metacognitive level—unlike the automatic reflexes and impulses associated with the emotional and behavioral systems—allows the individual to form conscious intentions (Beck, 1996), including, of course, the achievement of long-term goals. In goal attainment, the motivational and behavioral systems are activated and controlled through the conscious control system. In achieving remote (in time) goals, this system resolves conflicts by simply overriding the control of short-term consequences. This is accomplished through such strategies as ignoring unpleasant affect associated with sustained goal-directed behavior (e.g., mild fatigue) and rational responding to negative automatic thoughts (e.g., fear of failure). Such override is logically necessary whenever the automatic systems are programmed to respond to aversive (or positive) short-term consequences by selecting behavior inconsistent with the long-term intended goals.

A problem for continuing experimental research is how the correction of cognition (product) through reevaluation (metacognition) leads to improvement. One explanation is that the ES (the automatic cognitive level; Epstein, 1994) operates more reflexively and is intended to deal with certain general features of the environment (e.g., danger). Human biological adaptation is largely dependent on automatic (unconscious) processes. People are generally unaware of—and have little control over—most physiological responses to significant changes, such as temperature and other stressors. However, psychological and social adaptation is often enhanced by conscious cognitive operations, especially metacognitive processes. Again, the notion of "distancing" is equivalent to activation of the metacognitive level.

The metacognitive level operates to provide "fine-tuning" (cognitive tuning) for the ES. Thus, the RS is activated in those situations where feedback indicates the ES to be dysfunctional. When for whatever reason(s) the RS is not properly activated or functions inadequately, the cognitive therapist, in conducting cognitive therapy, provides assistance in its activation.

Another important mechanism for correction of distortions in cognitive therapy involves direct access to the ES through the use of imagery or fantasy. Clinical studies have shown that when reality distortions are incorporated into spontaneous fantasies, psychological disorder (e.g., anxiety) results (Beck, 1970b). Moreover, structured or "guided" fantasies have been shown to modify (correct) patients' overt behavior and to reduce maladaptive affect (Beck, 1970b). Guided imagery theoretically serves two functions: (1) It activates metacognitive (rational) processing, and (2) it is employed clinically to communicate directly with the experiential (automatic system) "in its own medium, namely fantasy" (Epstein, 1994, p. 721). Thus, the cognitive systems interact adaptively in cognitive therapy of psychological disorders.

## CONCLUSIONS

Experimental, clinical, and "common-sense" analyses support the formulation that conflicts between short-term and long-term behavioral consequences are psychopathogenic for a wide range of conditions seen in clinical psychological practice. Experimental and clinical studies supporting this thesis have been reviewed in this chapter. Regarding common-sense examples, most of us have directly experienced at least minimal conflict when faced with a choice between engaging in some behavior that has immediate positive consequences but probable negative delayed outcomes. Human behavior and adaptation are clearly influenced in part by cognizance of the temporal relationship between behavior and outcome.

To find personal examples of this phenomenon, we might simply ask our readers how their behavior would change if they had certain knowledge that their lives would end, say, within the next 3 months. Many readers would alter their behavior within this time period so as to maximize the (now redefined) "long-term" positive consequences. Depending on their values, some readers might spend more time with family members; others might renew professional or scientific efforts; and those who appreciate (but exercise appropriate control in regard to) certain culinary items might modify their diets in keeping with a 3-month time frame of consequences.

At a larger level of analysis, national budgetary processes often involve temporal-consequences conflicts. For example, when immediately expedient solutions are chosen, stressful negative consequences may be delayed but compounded to the point that coping resources (psychological and material) may not match long-term demands. Thus, societies must resolve this conflict by balancing outcomes so as to maximize positive consequences over the long term, taking into account resources available not only in the present but also in the future.

Several aspects of cognitive theory and metatheory have been described that provide a theoretical account of the resolution of temporal-consequences conflicts. Among these characteristics, cognitive theory not only attends to the role of environmental consequences in adaptation; it also explicates cognitive mediation and the operation of distinct cognitive systems. The brain of *Homo sapiens* has apparently evolved enough adaptability to provide not only for planning, selecting appropriate memories, and so forth, but also for overriding the more primitive cognitive–affective–behavioral patterns when these are perceived to be maladaptive. Thus, although learning can take place on the substrate of primitive patterns (as shown in the experimental manipulations of learning and behavioral theorists), humans can also learn at a "higher level" —one that is far more refined and, in many cases, more functional than the primitive operations designed for meeting emergency situations. This provides a theoretical explanation for the resolution of reinforcement (or temporal-consequences) conflicts. In mediating conflicts between short-term and long-term consequences, and especially in selecting behaviors that are adaptive in the long term, the conscious control system regulates behavior (see Beck, 1996).

# PART II

# COGNITIVE THERAPY AND PSYCHOTHERAPY INTEGRATION

# CHAPTER FOUR

# An Analysis of Integrative Ideology

In an important edited volume, Arkowitz and Messer (1984) brought together a number of experts to explore issues concerning the integration of psychoanalytic therapy and behavior therapy. The editors expressed their hope that this volume would "lead either to conceptual and clinical progress toward an integrated approach or to *a clearer sense of the obstacles involved*" (p. ix; emphasis added). In retrospect, it contributed to the latter rather than the former. Over a decade later, there is no integrated approach apart from the scientific (empirically validated) systems of psychotherapy. This state of affairs has led to a consideration of new approaches to integration, including the integration of basic cognitive psychological principles into clinical practice (Wolfe, 1994)—an approach endorsed by cognitive therapists (Beck, 1991a).

In this chapter, we present a critical analysis of the contemporary ideology of psychotherapy integration as a movement within the field of psychotherapy. Several basic, interrelated problems in the goal of developing new integrative therapies by combining elements of "pure-form" therapies are described: (1) the lack of scientific criteria (testable theory, empirical validity) for psychotherapy integration; (2) problems in definition and specificity; (3) the reliance on surveys to understand integrative practices; (4) confusion between formal and personal (idiographic) meanings of "psychotherapy integration"; (5) the inherently political nature of psychotherapy integration; (6) failure to appreciate the virtues of scholarly debates; (7) failure to invest in scientific theories; and (8) theoretical ambiguities concerning the common-factors approach to integration. Finally, we show how cognitive therapy provides some solutions to these problems, such as a common language for clinical practice and a technically eclectic approach made coherent by cognitive theory.

## PROBLEMS IN INTEGRATIVE IDEOLOGY

### The Absence of Scientific Criteria

There are three formal contemporary approaches to psychotherapy integration: (1) technical eclecticism, (2) theoretical integration, and (3) the common-factors approach (Arkowitz, 1991, 1992). "Technical eclecticism" in psychotherapy refers to the combination of clinical methods. As exemplified by the work of A. A. Lazarus (1967, 1989) and Beutler (1983, 1986), eclecticism is the selection of procedures from the various systems of psychotherapy on the basis of each procedure's demonstrated efficacy. By contrast, "theoretical integration" refers to the attempt to provide a synthesis of diverse theoretical systems. In other words, this type of integration—especially as manifested in the work of Wachtel (1977, 1987) and Prochaska and DiClemente (1982, 1984)—attempts to develop metatheoretical approaches to psychotherapy. Finally, the "common-factors" approach seeks to identify the core ingredients that therapies might have in common, with the eventual goal of developing new therapies based on these components (e.g., Goldfried, 1980). S. L. Garfield (1980,

1986), Frank (1973, 1982), and others view "nonspecific" factors in psychotherapy research as main elements of treatment (Omer & London, 1988).

Despite these formal ideological approaches, there have been few proposals for criteria for the integration of the psychotherapies. Yet such criteria would seem essential in explicating the meaning of "psychotherapy integration." Alford (1991) proposed two criteria (among others) by which to judge or define a psychotherapy system as integrative. The first criterion was that integrative therapy should incorporate all techniques and clinical procedures shown through outcome research to be effective in meeting the stated goals of psychotherapy. These would include attention to the therapist qualities and therapeutic relationship factors shown to be important in conducting successful therapy (see Beck et al., 1979, Ch. 3). The second criterion was that integrative therapy should reject the application of unproven therapies in cases where validated ones are available to meet the goals selected by client and therapist. Of course, if the unproven therapy were applied as part of an experiment, then informed consent would describe the nature of the study.

We would add to the two criteria above the stipulation that the techniques incorporated must be theoretically consistent with the therapy system appropriating the techniques. Since psychotherapy encompasses many aims, goals would include the outcomes collaboratively selected by the therapist and the psychotherapy patient. It would of course be necessary to test the efficacy of the intervention in the new therapy context.

As in the clinical practice of medicine, persons undergoing psychological treatments often show idiosyncratic response to standard approaches. A strategy found to be generally useful in alleviating symptoms of a specific disorder may be ineffective for a specific individual (see Beutler, 1983). Furthermore, advance matching of treatments to individual patient characteristics may prove impossible, because of the complexity of variables relevant to clinical practice. Empirical observation of responses as determined by homework exercises (rather than a set of decision rules) may prove to be a more reliable method for determining treatment strategies. Thus, a technically eclectic approach would appear desirable in order to make a variety of technical interventions available.

A central problem in delineating criteria for psychotherapy integration relates to the absence of theoretical integrity or coherence. Yet absence of theory may be necessary in order to promote the kind of openness valued by integrationists. However, without theory, can one sustain the criterion of empirical validity, since this criterion is considered (within scientific disciplines) to be a characteristic of a good theory rather than one of techniques? Of course, one response is simply to accept that certain techniques have been shown to work, and to disregard the questions of underlying theoretical process. The disadvantages of such an approach are elaborated below.

## The Absence of Definition and Specificity

Another problem concerns the interrelated issues of definition, specificity, and conceptual integrity. This particular conundrum faced by psychotherapy integration seems especially difficult within the common-factors approach. For example, the notion of the "therapeutic relationship" or "alliance" is the foremost common factor identified by those who believe in this approach (Grencavage & Norcross, 1990). Yet the notion of the therapeutic relationship as the vehicle for change (e.g., Arkowitz & Hannah, 1989) is typically presented in a nonspecific fashion. Indeed, lacking a theoretical context, the therapeutic relationship as a common factor becomes poorly defined, nonspecific, and unintelligible. In a word, it becomes (quite literally) a meaningless concept.

This is not true within the well-defined major systems of psychotherapy. In theoretical systems, the meaning of "therapeutic relationship" is consistent with the overall theory of therapeutic process. For example, in psychoanalysis the role of the therapist is seen as the maintenance of an impersonal (opaque or ambiguous) stance, so that interpersonal reactions of the patient are determined by (or reflective of) transference. Behavior therapists generally view the relationship as important to the extent that negative interpersonal reactions impede the implementation of behavioral strategies for change. Cognitive theory considers the "collaborative working relationship" to be important in allowing therapist and patient to work together to examine dysfunctional thinking and beliefs. Also, patients often reveal dysfunctional (distorted) conceptions of the therapist's behavior, so that cognitive distortions of an interpersonal nature (or content) may become the focus of treatment. Thus, a cognitive formulation of the "therapeutic relationship" would define this concept quite specifically to include the following: (1) a shared view regarding expectations of therapy; (2) session-by-session agreement on agenda; (3) agreement on the conceptualization of problems and the goals of therapy; and (4) the development of a common view between therapist and patient on the nature of the disorder or problem that led to the need for treatment.

## Surveys and Science

In a previous article (Alford & Norcross, 1991), surveys were cited that showed cognitive therapy to be the most popular system of psychotherapy chosen by self-designated "eclectics" for combination with other approaches (see also Arnkoff & Glass, 1992, pp. 679–681). Though this might be taken as evidence to advance the thesis of the present volume, surveys are merely tabulations of opinions held by those who are surveyed. They are useful primarily in determining what people may *think* about the practice of psychotherapy. Therefore, the scientific credibility of utilizing cognitive theory as a paradigm for integrative practice does not depend solely on the results of surveys.

Surveys do not replace the scientific process of testing those theories, or integrative paradigms, that may be most popular at a given point in history. Consequently, the fact that most practitioners (as contrasted with psychotherapy researchers) hold an "integrative" perspective is irrelevant to the question of the empirical validity, parsimony, and theoretical coherence of integrative approaches to treatment. As Robert Sternberg recently noted in another controversial context (over the book *The Bell Curve*), "I don't think science is done by majority vote" (quoted in Holden, 1994, p. 1811). The limitations of survey data in shedding light on integrative practices are considered next.

## Multiple Meanings of "Psychotherapy Integration"

Surveys have consistently found that the majority of psychotherapy practitioners describe their practice of psychotherapy as "integrative" or "eclectic" in nature (for a review, see Arnkoff & Glass, 1992, pp. 679–681). However, the precise meaning of such self-descriptors cannot be ascertained from the survey data available. Moreover, the distinction between formal (integration movement) models and personal (idiographic) models of integration has not been considered. Four possibilities are considered, as follows: (1) Most psychotherapy practitioners do not follow the theory or practice of any of the major systems of psychotherapy; (2) practitioners apply one (or more) of the formal contemporary models of integration; (3) psychoanalytic and psychodynamic practitioners are exploring alternatives because their faith in long-term approaches is decreasing; and (4) practitioners designate themselves as "integrative" because they integrate their own personal experience, personality, and knowledge into the clinical setting. (As shown below, we believe the third and fourth possibilities to be the most sensible interpretations of survey data.)

To take the first possibile interpretation, do the survey respondents (Arnkoff & Glass, 1992) mean to say that their clinical practice does not follow the philosophy, theory, and application (procedures, techniques, or strategies) of any of the established scientific systems of psychotherapy? Probably not. Indeed, surveys suggest that practitioners most commonly employ theoretical combinations that involve cognitive therapy—namely, cognitive and behavioral; humanistic and cognitive; and psychoanalytic and cognitive (Norcross & Prochaska, 1988). Thus, eclectic/integrative therapists do not appear to view integration apart from the established approaches to treatment.

A second possible interpretation of survey reports is that such reports indicate that practitioners subscribe to one of the formal contemporary models of integration: common factors, technical eclecticism, or theoretical integration. Again, this is unlikely; indeed, it would be a quite cynical interpretation of practitioners, since there is as yet no empirical validity associated with these formal approaches. The therapeutic efficacy of the contemporary approaches to psychotherapy integration is, in the words of Castonguay and Goldfried (1994), "more of a promise than a documented reality" (p. 167).

The third interpretation relates to the previous theoretical orientation of those who describe their practice of psychotherapy as "integrative" or "eclectic." Two independent surveys have concluded that most clinical psychologists calling themselves "eclectic" were previously psychodynamic or psychoanalytic (Arnkoff & Glass, 1992). This finding may reflect the decreasing faith in these particular approaches—and the search for a viable substitute—among psychoanalytic and psychodynamic practitioners (Norcross, Alford, & DeMichele, 1992).

A fourth and final interpretation of what many practitioners mean by describing themselves as "integrative" or "eclectic" is simply that they apply the various psychotherapies in a manner that integrates *their own personal experience, personality, and knowledge* into the clinical setting. This practice would appear consistent with developments in the philosophy of science, which suggest a sharp distinction between basic and applied science. For example, Manicas and Secord (1983) describe the distinction between the scientist and the clinician or technician as follows: "The former practices science by creating at least partially closed systems; the latter uses the discoveries of science, but . . . also employs a great deal of knowledge that extends beyond science" (p. 412).

## The Politics of Psychotherapy Integration

It is important to note that there are substantial differences between a psychotherapy integration movement and an integrative system of psychotherapy. The psychotherapy integration *ideology* (with which we as cognitive therapists differ) must be separated from the *goals* of integration (with which we are in complete agreement). The integration movement is characterized by all that makes up a political group, including such things as an "us" versus "them" mentality, a "party line," and vested political interests in promoting the agenda of the party. (Of course, to the extent to which the established systems of psychotherapy are not committed to testing their theories and therapeutic interventions, the same characterizations might apply as well to them.)

A number of ideological positions regarding psychotherapy integration have recently been articulated. Many of these challenge the principles that guide the continued evolution of the major scientific systems of psychotherapy, and argue for the replacement of the established approaches with "integrative" psychotherapy (see Alford, in press). Castonguay and Goldfried (1994) state the following positions: (1) "Acrimonious debates" within science are counterproductive (p. 159); (2) the improvement of traditional systems of psychotherapy depends on (or results from) a rapprochement with other systems (p. 161); and (3) those individuals who are involved in theoretical integration (compared to those who develop and test individual theories) have a "more complex and less biased" understanding of the etiology of psychological disorders (p. 161).

The challenges of psychotherapy integration to the established scientific (theoretically coherent and empirically validated) systems of psychotherapy have sometimes taken on a political tone. This issue has become apparent to writers both outside and inside the psychotherapy integration movement. For example, Andrews, Norcross, and Halgin (1992, p. 581) observe the following: "In much of the literature on psychotherapy integration, nonintegrative programs are portrayed as showing rigidity in the curriculum. . . . One difficulty with this account of obstacles is that it has a judgmental flavor, as evidenced by the use of words like *rigid* to characterize the opponents of integration." This political aspect of the psychotherapy integration movement has led A. A. Lazarus, one of the most distinguished pioneers of the eclectic/integrative approach, to conclude that "a state of even greater chaos now prevails. Instead of seeking unification, different schools of eclectic and integrative therapies seem to be proliferating" (A. A. Lazarus & Messer, 1991, p. 144).

## Discouragement of Constructive Scientific Debate

An inherent aspect of the evolution of any scientific discipline is vigorous intellectual debate regarding theories. Advancing, testing, and debating theories are all part of the process of science. Consider the following description of this process as it has occurred within the field of biological evolution:

An almighty dispute erupted, with anthropologists and bio-chemists criticizing each other's professional techniques in the strongest of language. . . . The debate raged for more than a decade, during which time more and more molecular evidence was produced. . . . Finally, in the early 1980s, discoveries of much more complete specimens of *Ramapithecus*-like fossils, by Pilbeam and his team in Pakistan and by Peter Andrews, of London's Natural History Museum, settled the issue. . . . Even diehard *Ramapithecus*-as-hominid anthropologists were per-suaded by the new evidence that they had been wrong and Wilson and Sarich had been right: the first species of bipedal ape, the founding member of the human family, had evolved recently and not in the deep past. (Leakey, 1994, pp. 7–8)

The theorists in anthropology and biochemistry involved in this acrimonious debate could have chosen to find a "middle ground" or an "integrative" position that might have satis-fied both groups. However, the quality of their theories did not allow such a solution. The respective theories were test-able and predicted contradictory observations. One side won the debate, and the other side lost. In the process, science advanced.

Contrary to this example of constructive scientific debate, contemporary integration movement ideology suggests that the reduction of "acrimonious debates" is a desirable goal in the development of psychotherapeutic approaches (Caston-guay & Goldfried, 1994, p. 159). In connection with the re-duction of debates, integrationists cite the virtues of integra-tion, which include the following: "open inquiry, mutual respect, and transtheoretical dialogue" (Norcross, 1990, p. 298); "an attitude of openness and exploration" (Arkowitz, 1991, p. 1); "an open attitude . . . open-mindedness . . . less biased understanding" (Castonguay & Goldfried, 1994, p. 159, 161); and a sense that "We are good—they are also good" (Norcross, 1988, p. 420).

Such statements as these refer in large part to the hy-pothesized virtue of "theoretical openness." For example, part of the mission statement of the *Journal of Psychotherapy Inte-*

*gration* (which began publication in 1991) is as follows: "The journal is devoted to publishing original peer-reviewed papers that move beyond the confines of single-school or single-theory approaches to psychotherapy and behavior change. . . ." Thus, there is the suggestion that the various established scientific systems of psychotherapy may be "confined" in their theoretical structures and clinical techniques. Such thinking is presumably thought to be associated with counterproductive debates, which are to be avoided. For example, editor Arkowitz (1992) writes: "In the single-school approach, the therapist *believes in the theory* on which the approach is based" (p. 262; emphasis added).

This is a fundamental misconception regarding the nature of theory, and is not the view of theory taken by cognitive-behavioral therapists and researchers. Fishman and Franks (1992, p. 161) note that "there is no single and invariant scientific methodology . . . [and] the belief in any form of science itself is no more than a belief." To take another example, "good theory, like good therapy, is merely a working approximation until better theory or therapy comes along" (Franks, 1984, p. 254). Or, as Francis Crick (1994) explains:

> You cannot successfully pursue a difficult program of scientific research without some preconceived ideas to guide you. Thus, loosely speaking, you "believe" in such ideas. But to a scientist these are only provisional beliefs. He does not have a blind faith in them. On the contrary, he knows that he may, on occasion, make real progress by disproving one of his cherished ideas. (p. 257)

The notion that therapists in "single-school" approaches rigidly believe in their own theories—except in the limited sense defined by Crick above—is incorrect. Indeed, to suggest otherwise is to underestimate those clinicians and researchers who apply and test the various scientific systems of psychotherapy (e.g., Emmelkamp, 1994; Greenberg, Elliott, & Lietaer, 1994; Henry, Strupp, Schacht, & Gaston, 1994;

Hollon & Beck, 1994). Even undergraduate students are taught the dictum that scientific theories are neither true nor false, but rather more or less useful for explanatory and predictive purposes. On the development of theories of the various anxiety disorders, the following has been written:

> No one perspective is likely to provide an adequate explanation of clinical anxiety but a combination of different approaches can help fit together the various pieces of the puzzle. It is essential that investigators recognize the limitations and nonexclusivity of their own perspectives as well as recognize the contributions emerging from other vantage points. . . . A variety of research studies using a number of different models is most likely to advance our knowledge of the causes and treatment of clinical anxiety. (Beck, 1985b, pp. 195–196)

Similarly, in theorizing on clinical depression, six different models have been advanced to be subjected to empirical analysis (Beck, 1987a).

## Absence of Investment in Scientific Theories

Related to the preceding problem, another erroneous belief within contemporary psychotherapy integration ideology is that investment in theories is counterproductive to the development of effective psychotherapy. Investment in theories has been mistakenly identified by psychotherapy integrationists as antithetical to scientific progress (Alford, in press). In discussing the further development of psychotherapy integration, Castonguay and Goldfried (1994) write that "this movement is not without barriers and obstacles, such as the therapists' investment in their personal theories" (p. 169).

Investment in theories is neither a barrier nor an obstacle, provided the theories are both testable and tested (Alford, in press). As Darwin once said, why would any scientist do anything if not to support or disprove a theory?

(cited in Eysenck, 1994, p. 479). Indeed, investment in theories has guided the development of the cognitive and cognitive-behavioral therapies (Hollon & Beck, 1994), as well as the other major psychotherapeutic approaches (e.g., Emmelkamp, 1994; Greenberg et al., 1994; Henry et al., 1994). Thus, one response to the concern over investment in theories is to consider the consequences (contributions of science) that have occurred over time as a result of advancing and testing scientific theories. Once again, Crick (1994) has explained the matter as follows: "That scientists have a preconceived bias toward scientific explanations I would not deny. This is justified, not just because it bolsters their morale but mainly because science in the past few centuries has been so spectacularly successful" (p. 257).

## Theoretical Ambiguity of the "Common Factors"

The final issue concerns arguments for developing new psychotherapies based on "common factors." Goldfried (1980) has suggested that a consensus may be achieved by focusing on a level of abstraction between the level of theory and the level of technique—a level he terms "clinical strategies." If empirical support for such clinical strategies should be obtained, he suggests that the term *"principles* of change" might then be substituted for "clinical strategies." He suggests two such strategies: (1) new, corrective experiences, and (2) offering direct feedback. This general approach is now considered to be one of the three major contemporary integrative approaches (Arkowitz, 1991, 1992).

However, this particular suggestion raises several questions. First, providing "new, corrective experiences" seems similar to the notion of a "therapeutic relationship," in that it is entirely tautological. ("Therapeutic relationship" is also frequently advanced as a common factor.) How can one test the idea that providing *corrective* experiences results in effective outcomes (corrections of presenting problems), since by definition they would do so? Moreover, Haaga (1986) correctly noted that to include all the meanings associated with "new experiences," only vague conclusions regarding psychotherapeutic process could be derived—for example, "For change to occur, something different has to happen" (p. 532).

Second, to offer direct feedback is clearly a cognitive process or intervention. Thus, it would appear to be a factor specific to those approaches that theorize the role of cognitive processes in psychotherapy. This is inconsistent with the concept of a "common factor." Third and finally, it is suggested that the term "principles of change" might replace the term "clinical strategies" if empirical support is obtained to support specific principles. However, *principles* would appear equivalent to *theories* in level of abstraction. Given this equivalence, there is then no tenable position from which to claim integrative theoretical neutrality.

As shown below (and in Chapter 5), cognitive therapy offers some solutions to the problems presented above, including a common language for clinical observations that is theoretically consistent yet broad in scope. In addition, the technically eclectic stance of cognitive therapy offers flexibility in clinical practice, while retaining the explanatory power (and testability) of a coherent scientific theory.

## SOLUTIONS OFFERED BY COGNITIVE THERAPY

### A Common Language for Clinical Observations

As noted by Alford and Norcross (1991), an important function for an integrative theory would be to provide a common language. A survey of 58 members of the Society for the Exploration of Psychotherapy Integration found that the absence of a common language was rated as one of the most severe impediments to psychotherapy integration (Norcross & Thomas, 1988). Cognitive therapy's constructs appear compatible with seemingly divergent perspectives, and may therefore assist those who are interested in integrating the various systems of psychotherapy.

The two most frequent contenders for a common psychotherapy language are ordinary language (e.g., Messer, 1987) and cognitive psychology (e.g., Kazdin, 1984; Ryle, 1982; Safran, 1984). Ordinary language may contain most of the necessary distinctions and connections found to be useful throughout the lifetimes of many generations. Similarly, cognitive concepts such as "schemas," "scripts," and "metacognition" have the potential for covering therapeutic phenomena observed by clinicians of varying orientations (Goldfried & Newman, 1986). Kazdin (1984, p. 163) writes that the concepts of cognitive psychology

> deal with meaning of events, underlying processes, and ways of structuring and interpreting experience. They can encompass affect, perception, and behavior. Consequently, cognitive processes and their referents probably provide the place where the gap between psychodynamic and behavioral views is least wide.

## Technical Eclecticism

The technically eclectic nature of cognitive therapy is one of its distinct characteristics (see Alford & Norcross, 1991; Arnkoff & Glass, 1992; Beck, 1991a). In this section, we elaborate on this particular aspect of cognitive therapy. We also show how cognitive theory, provides at least a partial solution to many of the problems of psychotherapy integration described above.

Those readers who are familiar with the basics of cognitive therapy know that cognitive therapy routinely combines techniques from a diversity of psychotherapies. Although most of the specific methods used in cognitive therapy have been divided into "behavioral" and "cognitive" categories (e.g., Beck et al., 1979), techniques are taken from other perspectives as well (Arnkoff, 1981; Beck et al., 1985). Indeed, any clinical technique that is found to be useful in facilitating the empirical investigation of patients' maladaptive interpretations and conclusions may be incorporated into the clinical practice of cognitive therapy.

However, the procedures used in cognitive therapy are not employed as isolated techniques. Instead, they represent the selection of methods in the service of a global clinical strategy consistent with the axioms of cognitive theory. A cognitive conceptualization of the individual patient determines the techniques selected (Persons, 1989).

Thus, cognitive therapy is highly eclectic, but not theoretically "neutral." On the differences between the application of techniques (technology) and a scientific system, Eysenck (1994, p. 479) has written the following:

> Science is essentially abstract, where technology is concrete. Science looks for laws, technology for rules. Science seeks for explanations, technology for applications. Each can aid the other, but there is an essential difference between them. This difference is related to the importance of large-scale, fact-based *theories.* (emphasis in original)

Techniques used in cognitive therapy are part of an overall conceptualization used to guide the practice of cognitive therapy of an individual case. One example is the use of role playing to activate "hot" cognitions associated with specific interpersonal events or situations (see Beck et al., 1985). In this example, a procedure employed in Gestalt therapy is employed in cognitive therapy. When it is used by a cognitive therapist, the goal is the activation of core schemas relevant to the person's dysfunction. Numerous other techniques besides role playing are used in this way (see Beck et al., 1985, 1990).

However, therapeutic procedures that may appear similar to an observer actually represent altogether different processes to therapists guided by different theoretical strategies. From a cognitive perspective, topographically identical techniques are functionally equivalent among diverse therapists only when such therapists share (and share with their patients) common rationales for their use (Alford & Norcross, 1991). Consistent with this point, Schacht (1984) has argued that a process resembling desensitization that occurs in dynamic therapy may resemble this process *topographically*, but not at the level of *strategy*. Like Messer (see A. A. Lazarus & Messer, 1991), he argues that context changes the meaning of any clinical technique: ". . . any given element acquires significance only within a structure of meanings and a system of functional relations. Thus, salt in one's soup is quite different from salt in one's gas tank" (Schacht, 1984, p. 121).

The technically eclectic nature of cognitive therapy has been described previously as follows: "By working within the framework of the cognitive model, the therapist formulates his [*sic*] therapeutic approach according to the specific needs of a given patient at a particular time. Thus, the therapist may be conducting cognitive therapy even though he is utilizing predominantly behavioral or abreactive (emotion releasing) techniques" (Beck et al., 1979, p. 117). Techniques can be selected from other psychotherapeutic approaches, provided that the following criteria are met: (1) The methods are consistent with cognitive therapy principles and are logically related to the theory of therapeutic change; (2) the choice of techniques is based on a comprehensive case conceptualization that takes into account the patient's characteristics (introspective capacity, problem-solving abilities, etc.); (3) collaborative empiricism and guided discovery are employed; and (4) the standard interview structure is followed, unless there are factors that argue strongly against the standard format (Beck, 1991a).

The cognitive approach may be integrated into the prevailing therapeutic technology already utilized in the treatment of a particular disorder or population. Cognitive therapy of couples' problems, for example, utilizes many of the standard marital therapy techniques (Beck, 1988b), and cognitive therapy with children incorporates techniques such as play therapy (Knell, 1990). In treatment of personality disorders, cognitive therapists may produce affective experiences, reactivate early memories, and role-play crucial past episodes. In cognitive therapy of panic disorder, panic attacks are induced in a manner similar to the behavioral techniques of flooding and implosion (Beck, 1988a).

An important discriminating feature of cognitive therapy is the structure of the interview, which includes an agenda, feedback, and homework assignments. The rationale of therapeutic interventions should be as clear to the patient as to the therapist. This format facilitates engaging the patient in the therapeutic process. This interview format is borrowed largely from behavior therapy: setting goals, breaking problems into specific components, defining procedures, measuring progress, and collaborating to develop homework assignments. The questioning format was derived originally from the "associative anamnesis" of Felix Deutsch, Carl Rogers's nondirective therapy, and Albert Ellis's Socratic questioning. The enactive, emotive strategies have been influenced by psychodrama and Gestalt therapy. Rational–emotive therapy has helped shape the testing or evaluating (but not challenging) of dysfunctional beliefs. The more manipulative strategies and other schools of psychotherapy are avoided when they conflict with the goal of patient as collaborator or personal scientist—an idea probably influenced by George Kelly. Thus, cognitive therapy is highly eclectic and does utilize techniques from other psychotherapies (Beck, 1991a). At the same time, however, it provides a paradigm for a coherent integrative practice.

## CONCLUSIONS

We have made a distinction between the contemporary integrative *ideology* (i.e., formal contemporary approaches to psychotherapy integration) and the aims or *goals* of developing a comprehensive system of psychotherapy. We have found numerous substantive problems in integrative ideology; at the same time, we believe that cognitive therapists share many (if not most) of the goals or aims of those who promote integration. Among the most important shared values is the intention to develop a proven scientific system of therapy. The criteria for such a theoretical system include theoretical consistency, parsimony, testability, and a comprehensive scope of applicability. In the chapter to follow, we turn our attention to these issues as we consider the status of cognitive theory as an integrative theory for clinical practice.

# CHAPTER FIVE

# Cognitive Theory as an Integrative Theory for Clinical Practice

Both the psychotherapy integration movement and the cognitive therapies have explicitly focused on integrating diverse approaches and knowledge bases into clinical practice (see Arnkoff & Glass, 1992). For example, part of the mission statement of *Cognitive Therapy and Research*, which began publication in 1977, is as follows: "[This] is a broadly conceived interdisciplinary journal. . . . It attempts to integrate such diverse areas of psychology as clinical, cognitive, counseling, developmental, experimental, learning, personality, and social." Similarly, the *Journal of Cognitive Psychotherapy*, which began publication in 1987, states: "This scholarly journal seeks to merge theory, research, and practice and to develop new techniques by an examination of the clinical implications of theoretical development and research findings. . . . Articles describing the integration of cognitive psychotherapy with other systems are also welcome." Compare these descriptions to that of the *Journal of Psychotherapy Integration* (which began publication in 1991): "The journal is devoted to publishing original peer-reviewed papers that move beyond the confines of single-school or single-theory approaches to psychotherapy and behavior change. . . ."

These three journals are obviously similar in their scope and intention to integrate diverse areas, including other systems of psychotherapy. However, one obvious difference is that a major aim of the *Journal of Psychotherapy Integration* is to move "beyond the confines of" the established theories and systems. In what follows, we argue that this position is untenable as a foundation for the development of comprehensive systems of psychotherapy. In order both (1) to move "beyond" the contemporary theories, and (2) to further the aim of developing a scientific approach to psychotherapy, psychotherapy integrationists must develop new theories of their own. Unfortunately for psychotherapy integration as an ideology, this is not a direction in which the movement seems interested. For example, the formal approach known as "theoretical integration" explicitly aims to combine theories rather than to develop and test new ones. As we have noted in Chapter 4, such an approach has not been shown to produce coherent and testable theoretical formulations.

## THE ROLE OF THEORY

The idea that scientific theories are intrinsically confining is questionable. A number of writers have addressed this important issue. The typical view of the nature of scientific theories (or laws) is expressed quite well in the following descriptions by J. Cohen and Stewart (1994): "Laws are not timeless truths. They are context-dependent regularities, and we bring out different laws by asking different questions" (p. 285); "Our prized laws of nature are not ultimate truths, just rather well-constructed Sherlock Holmes stories" (p. 435).

A system of psychotherapy cannot evolve as a scientific discipline without a coherent theory of psychopathology and therapeutic process. Moreover, the therapeutic efficacy (and maintenance) of a psychotherapeutic approach will depend in large part on providing a coherent theoretical rationale to patients. As Messer says (A. A. Lazarus & Messer, 1991): "A psychological procedure cannot be administered like a pill, but will be shaped by the language and framework in which it is couched. When we move from the biological sphere to the arena of social science, we enter the realm of human meanings" (p. 156).

To return to the *Journal of Psychotherapy Integration*'s aim to move "beyond the confines of" the established theories and systems of psychotherapy, there clearly is a better choice than escaping the bounds of theory altogether. By keeping in mind the tentative nature of scientific explanation and theorizing, one can avoid becoming "confined," and yet at the same time can develop and test coherent theories. Again, the fundamental pathway to progress in scientific endeavors would appear to be the development of theories that are both testable and tested. Thus, scientific theories are not the enemies of scientific progress; rather, they are the *results* of such progress.

Numerous writers have addressed the issue of the essential role of theory in psychotherapy (and psychopathology). For example, Eysenck (1994, p. 479) has articulated the importance of theory within the field of psychotherapy as follows:

> What separates science from technology? Poincaré put his finger on the difference when he said: "Science is built up with facts, as a house is built with stones. But a collection of facts is no more a science than a heap of stones is a home." Technology consists of isolated advances, but science is *organized knowledge*. Technology works; science tells us why it works and predicts new advances . . . our major concern should be with the creation and working out of a *scientifically valid* theory underlying our efforts. (emphasis in original)

Similarly, Bergin and Garfield (1994) write: "The absence of good theory is a problem. There is not much of the kind of conceptual coherence one would expect from an advancing scientific discipline" (p. 822). And Franks (1984, p. 254) cites Montaigne: "No wind blows in favor of a ship that has no direction." Franks points out that it is the nature of theory to provide a working approximation until better theory comes along, and adds:

> . . . this "coming along" is *not* a matter of chance. It is more likely to occur within the disciplined exploration of some theoretical framework than in either an eclectic pursuit of whatever happens to be around or a premature integration of two systems that, to my way of thinking, are clearly incompatible and best left, at least for the time being, to develop independently. (Franks, 1984, p. 254)

If this line of reasoning is correct, it raises the question of the criteria for good scientific theorizing—a topic to which we now turn our attention.

## CRITERIA FOR A SCIENTIFIC THEORY

A number of criteria have been suggested for evaluating scientific theories (see Liebert & Spiegler, 1987). Here, we consider the manner in which cognitive theory meets the criteria for a scientific theory, including its internal consistency, parsimony of explanatory constructs, testability, and scope of clinical application. We also consider how cognitive theory provides a paradigm for integrative clinical practice. In a later section of the chapter, we articulate the relationship between cognitive therapy and the psychotherapy integration approach known as "theoretical integration."

### Theoretical Consistency

As discussed in detail in Chapter 1 (and consistent with Popper, 1959), the formal statement of cognitive theory includes all the necessary and sufficient assumptions of the theory and forms the apex of the system. All theoretical statements may be derived logically from the axioms, which clarify and define the scientific theory. The requirement of internal consistency stipulates that the axioms must be free from contradiction. Moreover, Popper (1959) suggested that the axioms must be independent, so that no axiom is deducible from others within the system; that the axioms must be sufficient to permit the deduction of all statements belonging to the theory; and, finally, that the axioms must be necessary for derivation of the statements belonging to the theory. Clinical cognitive theory as presented in Chapter 1 meets these criteria.

## Parsimony

The second criterion is parsimony, of which there are different measures in cognitive theory. For example, one may evaluate the range of phenomena explained by the 10 axiomatic statements, and consider whether simpler formulations have been advanced to account for the same range or scope of observations. Here, we focus on one aspect of the parsimony criterion—namely, the manner in which cognitive constructs subsume those of other therapeutic approaches. This aspect has been termed the "common factors" of effective psychotherapy.

The common factors theorized by cognitive therapy are those that produce a positive change in the person's ability to obtain and process information relevant to successful adaptation to the environment (see Beck, 1987b). Cognitive theory stipulates that symptomatic improvement in the acute (Axis I) disorders is produced by deactivation of hypervalent schemas specific to a given disorder (such as depression, generalized anxiety disorder, or panic disorder). Moreover, evidence suggests that cognitive therapy produces enduring structural change, in addition to simply deactivating dysfunctional schemas. Thus, prevention of relapse in such disorders as depression or panic disorder is predicted by cognitive theory. Preliminary support for this prediction has already appeared, in that cognitive therapy of depression, compared to psychopharmacotherapy, lowers relapse probabilities (Hollon & Najavits, 1988).

Cognitive theory also guides the selection and timing of interventions. For example, techniques may be selected (1) to deactivate a hypervalent dysfunctional schema, (2) to activate and modify a chronic schema, or (3) to construct adaptive schemas. Also, it has been shown how the components of other therapies may produce change through cognitive restructuring (Beck, 1987b). Techniques from diverse systems of psychotherapy (cognitive, behavioral, psychodynamic, humanistic, and experiential) enable patients to disconfirm the basic dysfunctional beliefs embodied in the dysfunctional schemas. As is common in the case of depression, symptoms may also remit without therapy (Beck, 1967). Regardless of the approach to cognitive modification (direct or indirect), the dysfunctional beliefs that are activated during acute episodes of a disorder are no longer found when the episode is over.

In summary, the "common factors" of the psychotherapies are theorized to rely primarily on correction of dysfunctional cognitive content and processing. Cognitive modification can occur through a variety of procedures, including the therapeutic relationship, abreactive techniques, or explanation and interpretation. The most direct approach, however, involves an explicit focus on belief systems and developing coping strategies. The analysis of the therapeutic components and procedures of psychoanalysis, behavior therapy, and other systems of psychotherapy suggests one common factor—the modification of core beliefs or schemas (Beck, 1987b, 1991a). This perspective provides a parsimonious account of psychopathology and clinical phenomena.

## Testability: Hypotheses about Panic Disorder as Examples

To insure the scientific foundations of clinical cognitive theory (or any theory), the criterion of testability is probably the most salient of all the criteria considered here. A comprehensive review of the testable hypotheses of cognitive theory—including hypotheses regarding all clinical disorders that have been or could be subjected to experimentation—is clearly beyond the scope of this volume. However, in addition to the controlled outcome studies attesting to the efficacy of cognitive therapy (Hollon & Beck, 1994), cognitive *theory* has proven to be easily testable, as shown by the numerous studies designed to evaluate various hypotheses derived from it. The cognitive theory of depression (Beck, 1987a), for example, has generated several independent lines of experimental research (Haaga et al., 1991).

Hypotheses are readily derived from the cognitive theories of other disorders, such as panic disorder and the psychotic disorders, to which we turn our attention in Part III of this volume. Numerous hypotheses regarding cognitive therapy of psychotic disorders are included in Alford and Beck (1994) and Alford and Correia (1994), and these are not repeated here. In regard to panic disorder, specific questions and hypotheses consistent with a cognitive theoretical perspective are readily derived. The following detailed hypotheses, which may be subjected to empirical tests, are presented here as examples of how cognitive theory of a specific clinical disorder generates a wealth of ideas for research on psychopathology:

1. Catastrophic misperception of interoceptive cues occurs in panic disorder according to automatic (unconscious) as well as conscious processes. Panic patients are predicted to display this specific cognitive content during panic attacks (D. M. Clark, 1986).

2. Cognitive therapy of panic disorder is largely effective through the process of developing compensatory metacogni-

tive skills, which result in deactivation of these misperceptions or changes in patients' beliefs/schemas. Cognitive therapy, or any effective psychotherapy of panic disorder, may be found to work by means of this "common factor"—the development of controlled, deliberative information processing. Such processing will have the effect of reducing or eliminating the catastrophizing of sensations.

3. Decreases in "strength-of-belief" ratings in the fear or danger of physiological, psychological, or social consequences of panic sensations should parallel effective treatment of panic disorder. (One methodological point that must be noted is that researchers must be carefully trained in cognitive therapy, in order to identify the predicted processes [Beck, Newman, & Wright, 1989]. Given the often idiosyncratic nature of distortions in interpretation of physiological sensations, there may be no substitute for clinical skills focused precisely on uncovering the cognitive components responsible for activation of panic in individual patients [see Yeaton & Sechrest, 1981].)

4. Decreases in strength-of-belief ratings in the danger of physiological, psychological, or social aspects of panic sensations not only should parallel effective treatment of panic disorder, as suggested in hypothesis 3 above, but also should predict relapse. Additional analyses of the components of treatment are clearly needed, such as replications of the study by Craske, Brown, and Barlow (1991), which found cognitive restructuring to be more effective than relaxation at a 2-year follow-up.

5. Effective treatment will not be possible without improvements in these specific cognitive ratings, as suggested in hypothesis 3 above.

6. Conversely, effective treatment will always be observed whenever improvements are obtained in these specific cognitive ratings, suggested in hypothesis 3 above.

7. Reported decreases in strength-of-belief ratings made *during* naturally occurring or clinically induced panic episodes

should be especially powerful in predicting decreased severity of panic disorder.

8. Somatic sensations similar to those reported during a panic attack may still be reported subsequent to the successful elimination of panic disorder. However, these sensations are predicted to be rated or perceived as relatively innocuous after successful treatment.

9. The cognitive symptoms of panic disorder—thoughts of dying, of going crazy, or of doing something uncontrolled— are theorized to relate in a lawful manner to the physiological sensation symptoms. Specifically, at the phenomenological level there is predicted to be a perceived connection between a given panic patient's cognitive symptoms and the physiological symptoms listed in DSM-IV (American Psychiatric Association, 1994). In modern (cognitive) conditioning terminology, the physiological symptoms (i.e., shortness of breath or smothering sensations, dizziness, faintness, palpitations, etc.) are phenomenologically related to, or misrepresented as, *predictors* of catastrophic events. Since panic attacks are theorized to involve catastrophic (mis)representation or interpretation of the noncognitive symptoms, research should be directed toward determining at the phenomenological level whether the noncognitive symptoms are associated with the catastrophic themes of the cognitive symptoms.

10. Panic treatments that focus on reattribution of sensations should be more effective than procedures that simply include exposure to stimulus situations or sensations associated with panic. The basis for this hypothesis is that although exposure alone may frequently result in more adaptive associations (or predictions), it often fails to do so. (A study by Salkovskis and Clark, 1991, has found preliminary support for this hypothesis.)

11. Further research is needed to explicate the role of metacognitive processes in clinical disorders (see Flavell, 1984). Conscious awareness of cognitive processes/content in itself may be necessary but not sufficient as a corrective for

panicogenic schematic activity. Clinical cognitive research should be directed to identify the sufficient factors for adaptive cognitive reprocessing, once such processing has become the focus of attentional resources. The cognitive model would predict that the (theorized) panicogenic content is generally better changed through a combination of enactive and Socratic (guided discovery) procedures, rather than use of either alone. It would further predict the enactive or "behavioral" techniques to be effective *only* to the extent to which they modify the core cognitive configuration that has been implicated in panic disorder—namely, misattribution (guided by nonconscious mental structures and processes) of innocuous sensations.

## Comprehensiveness and Scope of Application

A central challenge of psychotherapy integration is to facilitate "the development of a comprehensive psychotherapy based on a unified and empirical body of work" (Norcross, 1986, p. 11). This criterion—scope or comprehensiveness— would appear to be a reasonable one for any theory or system of psychotherapy. For example, over 20 years have elapsed since Beck called for the admission of cognitive therapy into the "therapeutic arena" (Beck, 1976, p. 337), and well over 30 years have passed since he formulated the cognitive model of depression stimulated by research on dreams and other ideational material (Beck, 1961). In developing cognitive therapy, Beck (1976, p. 308) suggested the following criteria as necessary for any system of psychotherapy:

1. A comprehensive theory of psychopathology that articulates with the structure of the specific psychotherapy. The theoretical postulates should be related logically to one another, and the theory should be internally consistent, should be testable, and (within its own perspective) should possess reasonable explanatory power. (Added to those criteria are

[a] a tenable theory of personality, and [b] a theory of the process of change; Beck, 1991a.)

2. A body of clinically based knowledge and empirical findings that support the theory.

3. Credible findings based on outcome and other studies to demonstrate its effectiveness.

Comprehensiveness would appear to be a useful criterion, in terms of both the range of disorders to which it can be applied and the variables to which therapists attend. There is little controversy regarding the scope of application of cognitive therapy (Hollon & Beck, 1994). In addition to giving adequate attention to a wide range of variables implicated in the development and maintenance of psychopathology, cognitive therapy has been shown to be effective in treating numerous clinical psychiatric disorders: depression; generalized anxiety; eating disorders; substance abuse; obsessive–compulsive disorder; bipolar disorder; depression in HIV patients; avoidant and obsessive–compulsive personality disorders; paraphilias; posttraumatic stress disorder; multiple personality disorder (now dissociative identity disorder); hypochondriasis; marital problems; schizophrenia and other psychotic disorders; and others (Hollon & Beck, 1994).

### Criticisms of Cognitive Therapy's Scope

Despite the demonstrated scope of clinical cognitive theory and therapy, Coyne (1994) has recently raised this concern: "If cognitive theory rises to ascendency as *the* integrative theory, then the domain of integrative psychotherapy must shrink. Emotions and complex interpersonal processes within and outside the therapy session get downplayed or reduced to a matter of cognition" (p. 404). He continues by suggesting that cognitive theory construes interpersonal stressors entirely as products of biased or distorted judgment. Prochaska and Norcross (1994) raise a similar concern, as follows:

Cognitive therapies make the same mental mistake of many patients and many true believers—overgeneralization. . . . cognitive therapies conclude that nothing is awful or catastrophic. These overgeneralizations negate the tragic side of life and place a patient profoundly depressed by the death of a wife and three children in the same category with someone depressed over the loss of a promotion. (pp. 340–341)

Thus, there has been a failure to understand the multidimensional nature of cognitive theory and therapy. Given this situation, let us clarify specific aspects of cognitive therapy that have been the focus of misconceptions in integrationists' writings.

## Response to the Criticisms

In responding to these points, we return to the theory and metatheory of cognitive therapy as articulated in Chapters 1 and 2. The examples presented above suggest that cognitive theory ignores a set of variables that no serious system of psychotherapy could afford to ignore—that is, interpersonal and environmental variables. Over 30 years ago, Smith (1964) made an identical criticism: "There is an obvious denial of social reality which directly opposes, and is incompatible with, a pragmatic world view" (p. 151). This mistaken belief survives in the absense of support from either of the two major cognitive systems of psychotherapy. Indeed, both Beck and Ellis have made attempts to correct this misconception.

In response to the criticism by Smith (1964) noted above, Ellis (1965) explained his theory as follows: "We rational–emotive therapists do not in the least try (as Smith seems to think we do) to get the patient to deny that others can effect [*sic*] adversely. . . . They can easily, for example, maim him, kill him, put him in jail, fire him from his job, etc." (p. 109). He further stated: "I am not clear where Dr. Smith got this idea, since rational–emotive therapists do not dismiss *any* responses or events in the lives of patients . . . the rational–emotive practitioner, moreover, often agrees with his patients that their concern about hydrogen bombs, air pollution, racial injustices, etc. may be legitimate and helpful" (p. 111). Similarly, cognitive therapists have explicitly acknowledged that reality itself is often extremely *bad* (Beck, 1989); such an acknowledgment is essential, for example, in the cognitive therapy of cancer patients (Scott, 1989).

What does it mean to say that cognitive therapy reduces emotions and complex interpersonal processes to a matter of cognition? Presumably, the concern is that "cognition" in cognitive therapy may be equated with linear "thinking" or "calculation." Defined in this manner, cognitive therapy would suggest a much too simplistic theory to encompass the complex variables implicated in psychopathology (and effective psychotherapy). A review of some basic concepts—and of the definition of "cognition"—will help explicate this issue.

First, cognitive theory is a theory about the *role* (not the ontological exclusivity) of cognition in the interrelationships among such variables as emotion, behavior, and interpersonal relationships. "Cognition" includes the entire range of variables implicated in information processing, as well as consciousness of the cognitive products. Of particular importance in the present context, it includes consciousness of the objects/events that are known. According to this definition, cognition is a contextual, interactional construct. Its processing and phenomenological content are determined by (or responds to) environmental or contextual variables.

Cognitive theory suggests that internal and external phenomena impinging upon the human nervous system interact with that system, rather than that human cognition directly grasps (or "represents") reality. As noted earlier, Coyne (1994) has himself articulated the importance of analyzing not only "what is in the head," but also "how the head is in transaction with the interpersonal world" (p. 403). Thus, variables within the actual external environment and internal phenomenological experience are integrated. This theoretical position is taken in early formulations (e.g., Beck, 1964) as well as in more recent ones (Beck, 1991b). Certain basic theoretical constructs, such as schemas, are in one sense relational constructs. As we have noted in Chapter 2, Beck (1964, p. 562) cited English and English to define a cognitive schema as "the complex pattern, inferred as having been imprinted in the organismic structure by experience, that combines with the properties of the presented stimulus object or the presented idea to determine how the object or idea is to be perceived or conceptualized."

The concept "automatic thoughts" implicates both internal and external variables: "The relevant *beliefs* interact with the symbolic *situation* to produce the automatic thoughts" (Beck, 1991b, p. 370). Internal (phenomenological) and external (environmental) dimensions are integrated into the fundamental philosophical position and theoretical constructs of cognitive therapy. Through natural selection, cognition evolved to mediate between the environment and human organism. Thus, cognitive theory incorporates not only "information processing," but also ecological principles (see Safran & Greenberg, 1986).

To take one example that has also been mentioned in Chapter 2, "experiental" therapists convey their therapeutic approach by means of verbal (cognitive) constructs, not experiential ones. Humans convey or organize processes such as "behavior," "experience," "emotion," or "the therapeutic relationship" through cognitive constructs. Again, no other psychological function besides cognition provides this particular organizing function.

Since cognition includes consciousness of the knowing process itself along with the objects or events that are known, it is clearly a contextual, interactional construct. Put simply, human consciousness (cognition) intrinsically includes interaction with the environment. Through the design of homework experiments, the collaborative alliance in cognitive therapy focuses on (or "targets") events in natural environments.

One clear implication follows from what we have stated above: The assumption articulated by Coyne (1994)—that the domain of integrative psychotherapy will shrink if cognitive theory is taken as the integrative paradigm—is not correct. In cognitive theory, emotions and complex interpersonal processes within (and outside) the therapy session are not ignored or "reduced" to cognition. Cognitive therapists consider and treat the full range of emotions as such, interpersonal relationships as such, and a variety of other variables and stressors (Beck & Hollon, 1993, p. 91). The fact that reality is itself often extremely bad is confronted head on (Beck, 1989; Scott, 1989). However, in so doing, the cognitive therapist addresses the patient's sense of being trapped and hopeless. There is empathic understanding of the impact of the sad event, followed by the implementation of coping and problem-solving methods.

Discussions between therapist and patient in cognitive therapy include interpersonal and other environmental stressors related to the presenting problems, and *homework is designed accordingly.* Indeed, the personal meanings that are the central focus in cognitive therapy are typically found to relate to vital social issues, such as success or failure, acceptance or rejection, and respect or disdain (Beck, 1991b, p. 369). Cognitive therapy typically addresses emotional states, behavioral symptoms, expectations for improvement, experiences and meanings attached to experiences, and the likely positive or negative consequences of actions. Thus, cognitive theoretical formulations would appear flexible enough to incorporate a very broad scope of phenomena and clinical disorders within the fields of psychopathology and psychotherapy. The interpersonal relationship between client and therapist is of special importance (e.g., Beck et al., 1979, Ch. 3).

It should also be pointed out that the typical person who seeks psychotherapy does not expect the therapist to directly intervene and change the naturally occurring social and environmental context. Instead, those who seek therapy typically ask that the therapist assist in changing aspects of *themselves,* or they seek guidance in modifying their *reactions to* negative social and environmental contexts. Of course, a pragmatic approach will focus, as circumstances allow, on changing actual social or environmental conditions. However, changing personal reactions will probably remain the primary concern of psychotherapeutic interventions.

## COGNITIVE THERAPY AND THEORETICAL INTEGRATION

A number of issues relevant to theoretical integration have been addressed in Beck (1991a) and are elaborated here. These include (1) the extent to which cognitive theory has in the past incorporated other theoretical perspectives; (2) the integration of basic science such as cognitive science into clinical cognitive theory; (3) the question of whether current theories can add to the power of the axioms of cognitive theory; and (4) the strategy for insuring that the theory of cognitive therapy will not become a closed system like classical psychoanalysis, incapable of modification.

In developing the theoretical structure of cognitive therapy, Beck drew on other theories in addition to his own clinical observations. Cognitive therapy was in part derived from and in part a reaction against classical psychoanalysis (Beck, 1967, 1976). The emphasis on meanings, the role of symbols, and the generalization of reaction patterns across diverse situations were all derivative. However, the meanings were found to be available through introspection, and not to require the penetration or circumvention of a wall of repression in order to be elucidated. Other notions that were rejected included the predominantly motivational model, the idea of unconscious taboo drives defended against by mechanisms of defense, and the central importance attached to the psychosexual stages of development. Neo-Freudians such as Horney (and, to a lesser extent, Sullivan and Adler) contributed considerably to Beck's early formulations. Ellis's writings antedated Beck's and provided support for Beck's deviation from classical psychoanalysis. Novel interrelated theoretical constructs were developed, including cognitive vulnerability, cognitive priming, and cognitive specificity. Specific cognitive configurations (automatic thoughts and basic beliefs) were identified for the various clinical and personality disorders.

New theoretical constructs were tested as they emerged. Aside from the pioneering contributions of Ellis, cognitive therapy benefited minimally from the theories of other contemporary systems of psychotherapy, following the earliest formulations (Beck, 1964). Subsequent changes in theory evolved from cognitive psychology, social psychology, and evolutionary biology. Beck and others, taking a broader perspective on the origin and development of cognitive patterns, have traced them back to evolutionary survival principles (Beck, 1987a; Beck et al., 1985; Gilbert, 1989).

As cognitive theory continues to develop, emerging concepts in psychological disciplines such as cognitive psychology and social psychology will probably be of far greater importance than the influences of other schools of psychotherapy (Hollon & Garber, 1990) and the integration with theory of the other psychotherapy systems. The information-processing theory of personality and psychopathology (Beck, 1987a) is discordant with other systems of psychotherapy, so that attempts at a theoretical integration might result in logical inconsistency (Beck, 1991a).

Most theories of psychopathology and psychotherapy can add little to the explanatory power of cognitive theory. Moreover, there is a minimum amount of theory buttressing Gestalt therapy or Eriksonian therapy, for instance. To the extent that empirically validated principles are found within other systems, many of these have already been incorporated within cognitive formulations. Also, behaviorism as one of the more thoroughly validated approaches has now become quite different as a result of the "cognitive revolution"; cognitive constructs have replaced earlier notions.

Because many researchers continue to engage in systematic studies to test the conceptual models of cognitive therapy, cognitive theory is not very likely to become a closed system, as classical psychoanalysis has become. Theoretical progress in cognitive therapy will come not from fusion with other theories, but from clinical and experimental investigations of hypotheses derived from the formal axioms of cognitive theory. When a particular hypothesis does not hold up, the theoretical basis of the hypothesis will be modified accordingly. Again, since much of the theory of cognitive therapy is consistent with the basic psychological disciplines, the further evolution of clinical cognitive theory will probably come from experimental psychopathology and basic psychological research. Experimentation in cognitive or social psychology provides tests of the basic concepts of cognitive therapy. The other systems of psychotherapy can serve as sources of therapeutic techniques and procedures, as long as they are congruent with cognitive therapy (Beck, 1991a).

## CONCLUSIONS

In conclusion, we have focused here on the role of theory in a scientific system of psychotherapy, and on the manner in which cognitive therapy meets the criteria for a scientific theory. We have considered four criteria: (1) theoretical consistency; (2) parsimony; (3) testability; and (4) scope of clinical application. Although the theoretical framework of cognitive therapy does not incorporate the theoretical constructs of the other systems of psychotherapy, it does provide a broad (yet coherent) paradigm to guide clinical practice. Cognitive therapy provides a unifying theoretical framework within which the clinical techniques of other established, validated approaches may be properly incorporated. By assimilating proven techniques that are theoretically consistent with the cognitive perspective, cognitive therapy provides an integrative paradigm for clinical practice that is at the same time coherent and evolving.

# PART III

# COGNITIVE THERAPY AS INTEGRATIVE THERAPY: EXAMPLES IN THEORY AND CLINICAL PRACTICE

# CHAPTER SIX

# Panic Disorder: The Convergence of Conditioning and Cognitive Models

Although the possibility of integrating conditioning and cognitive models of panic disorder has recently been suggested (Davey, 1992; Rapee, 1991a; Rescorla, 1987, 1988), cognitive theory of panic disorder continues to be generally viewed as inconsistent with conditioning theory (e.g., Seligman, 1988; Wolpe & Rowan, 1988). Furthermore, and in accord with the reputed divergent theoretical formulations, the extant contemporary conditioning and cognitive *therapies* of panic are typically presented as distinct psychotherapeutic approaches (e.g., Barlow, 1988; Beck & Emery, 1979; Beck et al., 1985; D. M. Clark, 1986).

In this chapter, we advance a theoretical integration and suggest overlap between concepts derived from clinical observation and the basic psychological disciplines (Beck, 1991a, p. 193; Dalgleish & Watts, 1990; MacLeod & Mathews, 1991). (Staats, 1991, has used the term "unifying theory analysis" to describe this process of "rectifying the huge, untreated redundancy in psychology" [p. 905].) We clarify how cognitive theory of panic relates to contemporary conditioning theories. At the process level, theoretical divergence between conditioning and cognitive therapies of panic disorder is shown to be untenable.

## CONDITIONING AND COGNITIVE MODELS OF PANIC DISORDER

McNally (1990) has identified three contemporary theoretical perspectives on panic disorder: conditioning, personality, and cognitive. His analysis provides separate empirical and conceptual reviews for each of these models (for additional reviews, see Gelder, 1986; Michelson & Marchione, 1991; Rapee, 1987, 1991b). The present focus is on the conceptual overlap between two of these: conditioning and cognitive theories. In this section a brief history of each perspective is presented, and therapeutic exemplars of these perspectives are reviewed. It should also be noted that although genetic (and probably biochemical) factors have been implicated in panic disorder (e.g., Crowe, 1990; Klein, 1981), we are not dealing with these here.

### Conditioning Models

*Development of the Concept "Anxiety Conditioning"*

One of the first and most influential studies cited in support of conditioning models of anxiety was the case of Little Albert (Watson & Rayner, 1920). In this study, young Albert was found to exhibit fear to the presentation of a rat following several occasions of pairing the rat (CS) with a loud noise (UCS). The apparent conditioned fear generalized to similar furry objects, such as a rabbit.

Subsequent research found anxiety conditioning effects in humans to be limited and dependent on such variables as stimulus features, prior experience with CS and UCS, and characteristics of the learners (for reviews, see Chance, 1988; Marks, 1987b). For example, the concepts of "preparedness" (Seligman, 1971) and "prepotency" (Marks, 1987b) have been useful in calling attention to the role of evolutionary survival mechanisms (rather than a simple contiguous relationship between CS and UCS) in determining the operation of classical conditioning (see also Beck et al., 1985). Also, data suggest that developmental or maturational factors may determine which environmental stimuli produce fear responses at various chronological ages (Marks & Gelder, 1966). A comprehensive review of theoretical accounts of classical conditioning of anxiety is, of course, beyond the scope of the present chapter; however, the topic has been reviewed elsewhere by Marks (1987b, pp. 247–256) and Barlow (1988, pp. 222–225).

## Early Applications and Elaborations

Despite the limited work devoted to replication of the Watson and Rayner (1920) study, and despite failures to replicate their results when a different type of CS was used (see Marks, 1987b), the Pavlovian classical conditioning model was found useful by behaviorists in devising clinical treatments of anxiety. For example, after pairing relaxation with anxiety-evoking imagery, Joseph Wolpe theorized a "reciprocal inhibition" process in which anxiety responses are counteracted by relaxation responses (Wolpe & Rowan, 1988). Other learning theorists (such as Isaac Marks) have taken issue with Wolpe's account of the underlying mechanism of the conditioning process. To explain the observed therapeutic effects of behavioral treatments of anxiety, Marks (1987a, 1987b) has instead suggested the "exposure" principle as a common pathway to clinical change in the anxiety disorders. Marks has argued that since exposure alone is as effective as other treatments, "redundant components" such as relaxation may be eliminated (1987b, p. 458).

As noted above, conditioning theorists disagree regarding the relative merit of concepts such as "reciprocal inhibition" and "exposure" as therapeutic elements in the anxiety treatment process. However, there are basic similarities. In either case (whether reciprocal inhibition or simple exposure mechanisms are theorized), classical conditioning is seen as a reflexive, automatic process in which cognitive and experiential levels (deliberative, conscious levels) play little or no part.

This similarity among conditioning models—a conceptualization of anxiety based on notions of associative learning as an automatic, low-level, "mechanical" process—identifies noncognitive behavioral approaches to learning and is most relevant in the present context. Thus, the various debates regarding conditioning processes noted above are largely ignored, although interested readers may wish to pursue more fine-grained analyses on this topic, particularly as articulated by Marks (1987b).

### Contemporary Applications to Panic Disorder

Conditioning approaches to panic disorder and agoraphobia achieved greater prominence following the publication of successful controlled outcome (and follow-up) studies in the *British Journal of Psychiatry* (Gelder & Marks, 1966; Marks, 1971). Group therapy using the conditioning model was also found to be effective (Hand, Lamontagne, & Marks, 1974), and a controlled study by Marks et al. (1983) appeared in the *Archives of General Psychiatry*. In the 1983 study, 45 agoraphobics were randomly assigned to one of four treatment groups: (1) imipramine (doses to 200 mg/day for 28 days) plus therapist-aided exposure, (2) imipramine plus therapist-aided relaxation, (3) 25-mg placebo tablets (identical in appearance to the imipramine tablets) plus therapist-aided exposure, or (4) 25-mg placebo tablets plus therapist-aided relaxation.

Marks et al.'s (1983) overall results showed no superiority of imipramine over placebo (except at week 12 on one of seven measures), but they did show superiority of exposure over relaxation on measures of total phobia, one of the "global phobia" scales, anxiety–depression scores, and spontaneous panics in the last week. However, the superiority of exposure compared to relaxation was described as "slight," and the effect did not persist at a 1-year follow-up. The authors concluded, in line with other studies, that behavioral therapy is an effective treatment for phobias and panics (for a review, see Marks, 1987a).

Another important behavioral approach to panic disorder is the treatment developed by David Barlow and associates (e.g., Barlow, Craske, Cerny, & Klosko, 1989). A conceptual review of Barlow's approach to treatment of panic disorder shows that he has incorporated cognitive as well as conditioning formulations. Treatment elements, for example, include applied progressive muscle relaxation, exposure, and "cognitive restructuring" (Barlow et al., 1989). Although Barlow has incorporated both cognitive and behavioral approaches, he explicitly terms this approach a "behavioral treatment."

Thus, the theorized mechanisms of action of Barlow's behavioral model are not made explicit. The "cognitive restructuring" component is employed as a *technique* only. That is, this component does not appear to be conceptualized in terms of the goal of therapy and the theoretical mechanism of therapeutic change around which individualized treatment strategies are built (as in Persons, 1989); rather, it is utilized in a manner that A. A. Lazarus (1967) has termed "technically eclectic." In this context, it is not explicated how cognitive restructuring relates to behavioral theory. To be grounded in behavioral theory, an intervention would have to be derived from basic learning experiments and extrapolated to clinical intervention (Kazdin, 1978).

Rachman (1990) has stated "A verdict on the efficacy of conditioning therapy must await (additional controlled) clinical trials, but there is sufficient evidence about the effects of cognitive therapy to permit a preliminary evaluation" (p. 144). Regarding the question of the clinical status of pure conditioning therapies, one recent study found simple exposure (a behavioral procedure) to be ineffective in reducing panic when focus on misinterpretation of bodily sensations was not included (Salkovskis & Clark, 1991). Similarly, Barlow's work has shown the greater efficacy of cognitive therapy components. For example, an analysis of treatment components showed that cognitive restructuring controlled panic attacks more effectively than did progressive muscle relaxation, both at posttreatment and at a 2-year follow-up (Craske et al., 1991); perception of vulnerability is associated with panic attacks (Rapee, Telfer, & Barlow, 1991); and, consistent with cognitive theory (which specifies misperception of somatic stimuli or sensations), the most frequently reported stressors reported in initial panic attacks are somatic in nature (Craske, Miller, Rotunda, & Barlow, 1990).

## Cognitive Models

### Early Cognitive Studies

The intellectual antecedents of the cognitive approach to panic (and other emotional disorders) have a long history (see R. S. Lazarus, 1991a). In an article on Morton Prince, founder of the *Journal of Abnormal Psychology*, Oltmanns and Mineka (1992) suggest the value of considering the historical foundations of contemporary formulations of psychopathology. Oltmanns and Mineka (1992, p. 608) show how, in a case study of panic disorder, Prince invoked the notion of preconscious cognitive processing in a manner similar to the cognitive elements of Barlow's approach and to the contemporary approaches of

Beck and Clark (see below). However, the practical implications of such formulations were largely dependent upon development of the cognitive approaches to clinical treatment. Indeed, cognitive therapy has given particular attention to the treatment of panic disorder (Beck, 1988a; Beck & Emery, 1979; Beck et al., 1985; Beck & Greenberg, 1988; Beck, Laude, & Bohnert, 1974; Beck, Sokol, Clark, Berchick, & Wright, 1992; D. M. Clark, 1986; D. M. Clark et al., 1992; Salkovskis & Clark, 1986, 1990).

An early cognitive study of panic disorder, published in the *Archives of General Psychiatry*, was conducted by Beck et al. (1974). The main focus was on discovering the relationship between cognitions and anxiety. At the time of this study, DSM-II was the classification system used for the diagnosis of mental disorders. Anxiety neurosis was defined by DSM-II as follows:

> This neurosis is characterized by anxious over-concern *extending to panic and frequently associated with somatic symptoms.* Unlike Phobic Neurosis (q.v.), anxiety may occur under any circumstances and is not restricted to specific situations or objects. This disorder must be distinguished from normal apprehension or fear, which occurs in realistically dangerous situations. (American Psychiatric Association, 1968, p. 39; emphasis added)

In this study, Beck et al. (1974, p. 320) analyzed the ideational content of 32 anxiety patients, and found that (1) these patients had frequent thoughts and images relevant to the theme of danger, and (2) the hypothesized ideation (danger themes) was temporally connected to anxiety and was involved in the arousal and intensification of the anxiety. All but 2 of these 32 patients described acute anxiety attacks, whose "triggering stimuli" fell into three categories: *social*, *physical*, and *psychological* catastrophe.

Beck et al. (1974, p. 324) also described how the anxious patients differed from normal individuals by misperceiving innocuous situations as dangerous, and by persevering in thoughts or images about being physically or psychologically injured. Furthermore, a diathesis–stress model was advanced, as follows: "the model stipulates that as a result of certain kinds of stress impinging on a person's vulnerabilities, his concepts (schemata) relevant to danger become activated. These 'danger' schemata become prepotent and preempt the cognitive organization" (Beck et al., 1974, p. 324).

More detailed elaborations of the cognitive theory and therapy of panic disorder were subsequently published. For example, Chapter 6 of Beck's (1976) book, entitled "The Alarm Is Worse Than the Fire," elaborated on the notion of the vicious panic cycle (see especially pp. 149–151, the section "Spiraling of Fear and Anxiety"). Of particular relevance to contemporary formulations and theoretical integration are the description of fantasied "catastrophic consequences" identified in a college instructor who came to a hospital emergency room complaining of panic (p. 148), and the discussion of "stimulus generalization" and the involuntary fixation of attentional resources in panic disorder (p. 152). In addition to development of cognitive theory, a number of outcome studies have been conducted to assess the empirical validity of the cognitive treatment approach (e.g., Beck et al., 1992; D. M. Clark et al., 1992; Sokol, Beck, Greenberg, Berchick, & Wright, 1989).

## Convergence between Cognitive Models

Considerable attention has been focused on contemporary cognitive models of panic disorder, including the approaches articulated by Beck et al. (1985) and by D. M. Clark (1986). (According to an analysis of the *Social Sciences Citation Index* and *Science Citation Index* [E. Garfield, 1992], the Clark paper was the second most frequently cited article in all psychological journals from 1987 to 1991.) According to Clark's model, the essence of panic disorder is catastrophic misinterpretation of certain bodily sensations; that is, normal anxiety responses (such as palpitations) are perceived as much more dangerous than they really are. In this model, when internal or external stimuli are perceived as threatening, apprehension increases, and this results in physical sensations that are interpreted as catastrophic (see D. M. Clark, 1986; D. M. Clark, Salkovskis, & Chalkley, 1985).

Clark's model is consistent with Beck et al.'s theory (D. M. Clark, 1986, p. 462, footnote). A comparison of the two suggests an identity of conceptualizations, even though somewhat different words are used. Beck et al. (1985) describe the development of panic as follows:

> In many cases, the progression to a panic attack starts with a period of "tension" stemming from life problems. . . . At some point in the progression of a specific panic attack, symptoms intensify beyond the person's capacity to discount them or to function effectively. Her [sic] interpretation of sudden uncontrollable symptoms as signs of impending physical or mental disaster then accelerates the process until a full-blown panic occurs. (p. 136)

In Beck et al.'s theory of panic disorder, panic starts with some type of experience that the individual cannot attribute to something normal and that has for this individual the earmarks of an abnormal phenomenon. Therefore, there is a pathological attribution to the aberrant physical, affective, or psychological symptom (faintness, anger, disorientation). Schematic (meaning) processing occurs in which events are interpreted in terms of vulnerability schemas. Then comes the automatic content-specific faulty attribution. (Note how aspects of the two models overlap: "Catastrophic misinterpretation" [D. M. Clark, 1986, p. 462, footnote] and "interpretation of symptoms as signs of impending physical or mental disaster" [Beck et al., 1985, p. 136] or fantasied "catastrophic consequences" [Beck, 1976, p. 148] are equivalent.) This faulty attribution is framed in the form of a fear, "imminent danger," which then leads to anxiety.

At this point, the fear mode is activated within cognitive, affective, and motivational–behavioral systems. However, there is still no panic attack. It is only at the next point, where the individual's attention is fixed on (1) the physical, affective, or psychological symptoms and (2) the dire consequences, that the person begins to get into a panic attack. But it is not considered a real panic attack until the vicious cycle has been established and the anxiety and aberrant sensations escalate (see Figure 6.1, "PANIC BEGINS HERE"). The vicious cycle consists of the increasing anxiety's being "read" as confirmation of there being an internal disaster of some type. Thus, Beck and colleagues' theory of panic disorder incorporates the cognitive principles of unconscious (automatic) cognitive processing, the "vicious cycle," transfixed attentional resources, and cognitive content specificity.

### Access to the Unconscious

In cognitive therapy of panic, the patient learns to identify physiological sensations and negative automatic thoughts associated with the sensations. Once this has occurred, the patient is able to gain a sense of distance or objectivity regarding fearful thoughts. Baumbacher (1989) has presented a similar theoretical formulation regarding the role of "signal anxiety" in the etiology of panic disorder. Baumbacher conceptualizes signal anxiety as "a subjective experience that may be misperceived or not perceived for multiple reasons" (1989, p. 75), and elaborates the manner in which this misperception, or lack of perception, may lead to panic. Cognitive therapy of panic disorder is designed to enhance the patient's sensitivity to (and realistic interpretation of) normal physiological responses or sensations associated with anxiety. If misperceived, such responses can escalate via catastrophic misinterpretation

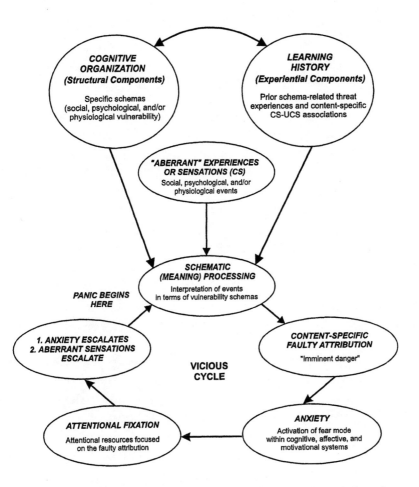

FIGURE 6.1. Cognitive and conditioning components of panic disorder.

in a "vicious cycle," leading to panic. Likewise, if the relevant physiological sensations and associated cognitions (referred to by Baumbacher, 1989, as "signal anxiety") are not consciously perceived, symptoms may escalate to the point of panic (Alford, 1993a; Alford, Beck, Freeman, & Wright, 1990). Thus, it is correct to say that cognitive therapy aims to make conscious certain processes that are initially unconscious.

## THE CONGRUENCE OF CONDITIONING AND COGNITIVE MODELS

The constructivist perspective of mainstream cognitive therapies is consistent with the implicit position of classical conditioning models, although this consistency has not yet been explicitly addressed by clinical conditioning theorists. The central conditioning concepts include conditioned and unconditioned stimuli (the CS and UCS) and conditioned and unconditioned responses (the CR and UCR). Implied in the theorized process of "unlearning" anxiety responses (through reconditioning techniques such as simple exposure or relaxation paired with anxiety) is the notion that such responses (constructions) do not match the demands of the person's environment (realism). Broadly conceived, the two perspectives agree that maladaptive anxiety such as panic attacks represent (1) disordered behavioral or cognitive activities of the person ("maladaptive responses" in conditioning theory, or "faulty constructions" in cognitive theory), in relation to (2) an actual environmental situation ("stimulus situations" in conditioning theory, or "reality" in cognitive theory).

Furthermore, there is a similarity between the central theoretical constructs of the two perspectives. The CS-UCS pairing that is theorized to lead to a maladaptive anxiety response is analogous in cognitive theory to an association between *sensations* (CS) and the interpretation of these as representing *imminent danger* (UCS). Specific idiosyncratic sensations (CS) automatically or reflexively activate the cognitive content "imminent danger" (UCS) (see Kreitler & Kreitler, 1982), and it is this repeated automatic associative processing that leads to the vicious cycle. Davey (1992) would add that the CS-UCS association is mediated by expectancy, and that the cognitive representation and evaluation of the CS (rather than the CS in itself) are what determine the anxiety response. This position is entirely consistent with cognitive theory (see Davey, 1992).

## Contemporary Conditioning Theory

Much of classical conditioning theory (e.g., Dickinson, 1980; Mackintosh, 1983) appears complementary to the cognitive learning perspective from which misattribution theory is derived. For example, unlike the earlier perspective that panic develops simply when "panic anxiety become[s] conditioned to contiguous stimuli" (Wolpe & Rowan, 1988, p. 446), contemporary Pavlovian conditioning "emphasizes the information that one stimulus gives about another. We now know that arranging for two well-processed events to be contiguous need not produce an association between them; nor does the failure to arrange contiguity preclude associative learning" (Rescorla, 1988, p. 152).

However, contemporary models of conditioning have yet to find their way into clinical formulations (Reiss, 1980). Siddle and Remington (1987) have stated that "the approach to Pavlovian conditioning adopted by many of those interested in experimental psychopathology involves a model of conditioning that has been rejected by many animal learning theorists for the past 20 years" (p. 139). Of particular relevance is the neglect of specific conditioning phenomena (e.g., postconditioning revaluation, blocking, sensory preconditioning) that support the role of cognitive processes in even the most simple learning paradigms (Kreitler & Kreitler, 1982), thus challenging CS-UCS contiguity theory (see Davey, 1987b, 1992; Siddle & Remington, 1987).

Evidence for inattention to current formulations is found in an article by Wolpe and Rowan (1988), which explicitly presents cognitive theory of panic disorder as inconsistent with conditioning theory, overlooking numerous contemporary empirical findings and theoretical developments in Pavlovian conditioning (e.g., Davey, 1987a; Dickinson, 1980, 1987; Mackintosh, 1983; Reiss, 1980; Rescorla, 1988). In this exemplar of noncognitive behavioral theorizing in this area, Wolpe and Rowan (1988) assume contiguity to be necessary and sufficient to create an association between the two events of interest (i.e., physiological stimuli and panic). Yet studies in Pavlovian conditioning have shown this to be an inadequate explanation for conditioning (Brewer, 1974; Davey, 1987a; Eifert & Evans, 1990; Mackintosh, 1983; Martin & Levey, 1985; Rescorla, 1988; Testa, 1974).

To take an example directly applicable to the cognitive theory of panic disorder, contemporary (cognitive) Pavlovian animal models address the observation that the CR can be modified by manipulating the present *evaluation* of the UCS (Holland & Rescorla, 1975; Holland & Straub, 1979; Rescorla & Holland, 1977). When Holland and Rescorla (1975) had their subjects conduct "postconditioning revaluation" procedures on the UCS following conditioning to a CS (e.g., reducing palatability of the food UCS through associating it with illness), they found responses to the CS to be inexplicably affected (see also Davey, 1987b; Revusky, 1977). Findings from such procedures have led researchers to postulate the presence of cognitive variables (e.g., memories) that facilitate prediction of the UCS by the CS; the simple operation of mechanistic S-R reflexes is no longer assumed (Davey, 1987b; Holland & Straub, 1979; Rescorla & Holland, 1977). Thus, conditioning process and cognitive process theories now appear indistinguishable (see also Rapee, 1991a).

## Phenomenology of Panic Attacks

According to the contemporary model of Pavlovian conditioning, conditioning involves "the learning of relations among events so as to allow the organism to represent its environment" (Rescorla, 1988, p. 151; see also Davey, 1987a, 1987b; Dickinson, 1980, 1987; Mackintosh, 1983; and Rescorla, 1988). This view is conceptually identical to the cognitive perspective (Beck et al., 1985; Beck & Greenberg, 1988).

The theoretical reformulation of conditioning to reflect cognitive processes has been applied to both operant and classical conditioning phenomena (see Rescorla, 1987). (Regarding operant [instrumental] *human* conditioning, cognitivists would observe that Skinner's concept of reinforcement might in this context be better conceptualized in terms of expectations for, and subsequent evaluations of, the consequences of actions.) A comparison of these apparently divergent areas of research (conditioning vs. the cognitive model) finds them to have common philosophical assumptions, a shared emphasis on an empirical level of analysis, and theoretically identical explanatory constructs (see Beck, 1970a). Cognition, or learning, is viewed as the process of representing complex relations among events so as to facilitate adaptation to changing environments (Beck et al., 1985; Rescorla, 1987, 1988).

Cognitive theorists simply seek to obtain a more complete picture of this representation (learning) through attention to the content of idiosyncratic, phenomenological perceptions of relationships among events. The phenomenological approach is a core component of cognitive theory in general and of the cognitive theory of panic disorder in particular. By contrast, classical conditioning models focus on an observer's view of relationships among events. Possible idiosyncratic perceptions of such relationships, and their qualitative content or meaning for survival, were not addressed in the early conditioning models.

Again, the cognitive theory of panic disorder hypothesizes specific cognitive content—that is, catastrophic misinterpretation of physiological sensations associated with normal response to anxiety (Beck et al., 1974, 1985; Beck & Greenberg, 1988; D. M. Clark, 1986; Hibbert, 1984), escalating in a "vicious cycle." Etiology is described in terms of distorted information processing (Beck, 1976; Beck et al., 1985), or, in contemporary Pavlovian conditioning terms, (mis)representation of relations among events (see Rescorla, 1988). However, cognitive theory increases the specificity of this explanation by hypothesizing the precise nature or *content* of such (mis)representation (e.g., rapid heart rate = "heart attack") and its importance in understanding the etiology of panic response (Beck & Greenberg, 1988). Researchers in basic psychological science, such as R. S. Lazarus (1991c), have recently noted the importance of such a phenomenological perspective in understanding emotional response.

Although "external" or "public" variables, which are traditionally the focus of classical conditioning paradigms, are not negated, cognitive theory does emphasize "internal" factors (i.e., misattribution). In Pavlov's original work with nonhumans, focus on such internal events was impossible (Pavlov, 1927). However, in subsequent conditioning studies with humans, the focus has shifted to include cognitive processes (Davey, 1987a). Therefore, the fact that phenomenological data, or "private" behaviors (Skinner, 1963), constitute a focus of cognitive research on panic does not indicate incompatibility between the cognitive and conditioning interpretations. Rather, the cognitive perspective simply attends to both levels of analysis—the physiological level (e.g., bizarre stimulus events, idiosyncratic sensations associated with anxiety) and the psychological level (catastrophic misinterpretation)—in the cognitive model of panic.

## Cognitive and Conditioning Processes in Panic Disorder

It has been evident for some time that the cognitive and behavioral psychotherapies have much in common (see e.g., Beck, 1970a; Michelson & Marchione, 1991). However, advances in basic psychological science have only recently provided evidence consistent with the convergence of mechanisms of action, or therapeutic processes, between these two approaches (Rapee, 1991a; Rescorla, 1987, 1988). The therapeutic processes that operate in both conditioning and cognitive therapies include the modification of dysfunctional thinking; durable improvement theoretically results from the modification of dysfunctional beliefs. (The specific content of thinking (and beliefs) and disordered cognitive processes thought to be implicated in the various clinical syndromes have been described previously; see Beck, 1976.) Both thinking and belief modification may be understood as regulated by the three cognitive systems or levels of cognition, as set forth in theoretical axiom 9 in Chapter 1—and elaborated in Chapter 3—of this volume.

The central question regarding cognitive versus behavioral treatments of panic disorder would seem at this point to be more theoretical than technical in nature. (Of course, answers to the theoretical questions will obviously then direct future technical advances.) The fact that the efficacy of cognitive therapy of panic has now been settled leads naturally to the next question—that is, how to explain the effective treatment theoretically (Sargent, 1990). Clinical cognitive theory stipulates that the underlying processes are cognitive in nature (Davey, 1992). The successful treatment of panic disorder (and *maintenance* of treatment gains; e.g., Hollon, DeRubeis, & Seligman, 1992) depends on concomitant surface and deep structural cognitive changes, whereby the person becomes more of an empiricist/realist.

## Postconditioning Revaluation

In "Contemporary Conditioning Theory" above, the experimental conditioning phenomenon "postconditioning reevaluation" has been mentioned. Clinically, postconditioning reevaluation of the UCS has a direct analogue in the cognitive therapy of panic disorder. As Beck (1992) has observed, patients who come to cognitive therapy are operating with their reflexes geared to both conscious and nonconscious processing. (Theoretically, there are several information-processing systems in operation simultaneously.) Cognitive therapists operate through the conscious part of the apparatus; that is, they try to strengthen the conscious part, so that it gets greater leverage or greater control over the nonconscious information processing. The aim of treatment is to correct the nonconscious processing, which tends to be global and undifferentiated. In the specific context of cognitive therapy of panic disorder, patients are trained to *consciously* reevaluate their responses to somatic stimuli. They learn to experience such stimuli, to reevaluate this experience, and to make the determination that there is no threat (see Beck, 1992).

In cognitive therapy, the panic patient is trained to reevaluate the specific physiological sensations (conceptualized as the UCS by conditioning theorists; e.g., Seligman, 1988; Wolpe & Rowan, 1988) that are misinterpreted as signaling imminent catastrophe (Beck & Greenberg, 1988; D. M. Clark, 1986; Sokol et al., 1989). As in the nonhuman conditioning studies cited above, the CR (panic response) triggered by the CS (in-session panic induction procedures; e.g., hyperventilation exercises) has been found to be affected or modified through revaluation of the UCS. Thus, revaluation of the UCS corresponds to the cognitive therapy procedure of teaching "rational responses" to the presence of specific physiological sensations similar to those of spontaneous attacks.

This is an interesting point of convergence between the cognitive and contemporary conditioning theories of panic disorder. In this case, the identified similarity is between animal conditioning phenomena and the central theoretical construct (and clinical intervention) of the cognitive therapy of panic disorder (Alford et al., 1990; Beck & Greenberg, 1988; Sokol et al., 1989). Although postconditioning revaluation theory in classical conditioning has to date been based solely on animal research (Holland & Rescorla, 1975; Holland & Straub, 1979; Rescorla & Holland, 1977; Revusky, 1977), the noted similarity suggests some degree of continuity between animal models and human behavior (see Davey, 1987b).[1]

## Temporal Primacy of Cognition

Several points concerning temporal primacy and cognitive causation are briefly reviewed here. Recent studies have assessed panic patients' experiences preceding panic attacks, including an empirical study by Argyle (1988) and a carefully controlled individual-subject analysis by Margraf, Ehlers, and Roth (1987). In the Argyle (1988) study, 77% of panic disorder subjects reported panic attacks following anxiety-provoking thoughts alone, without in the presence of phobic situations (p. 263). Margraf et al. (1987) found that providing the subject with false information (that her heart rate had suddenly increased) led to an unequivocal spontaneous panic attack (Margraf et al., 1987). The observed effects of information distortion are consistent with the cognitive model and provide a well-controlled case of how learning (wrongly) of a potentially threatening circumstance can lead to panic. Finally, Kenardy, Evans, and Oei (1988) analyzed naturally occurring panic during *in vivo* exposure. They obtained both cognitive and physiological measures of panic, and concluded

---

[1]Admittedly, this point of analogy is limited by the problem of unambiguous identification of the UCS and the UCR in theoretical formulations that posit Pavlovian interoceptive conditioning in panic disorder (e.g., Seligman, 1988; Wolpe & Rowan, 1988). McNally (1990) has delineated how the laboratory experiments on interoceptive–exteroceptive conditioning refer to empirically distinct and measurable events. Yet, in the conditioning models of panic, such clarity is not apparent (see McNally, 1990, p. 406). Perhaps a redefinition of UCS and CS in the context of panic disorder is necessary, as follows: The UCS is a stimulus that for a specific person has an innate cognitive association with *imminent* danger; the CS is a stimulus that has acquired such an association. Such definitions may better direct efforts to devise measurements consistent with contemporary conditioning formulations (as in Davey, 1992).

that specific cognitive processes ("catastropic cognitions") and physiological arousal are both necessary to panic onset.

Yet panic theoretically involves reciprocal influence among variables. These include physiological changes or psychosocial threat, and a cognitive component of specific content, which escalates symptoms in a "vicious cycle." The theorized panicogenic cognitions are intrinsic components of panic; sensations precede, accompany, and follow such cognitions.

Multiple systems are affected in panic disorder—affective, cognitive, behavioral, physiological—and, in fact, the panic syndrome consists of the activation of all these systems. The "billiard ball" analogy of causality (articulated initially by Newton) is obviously inadequate in this context (cf. White, 1990). Bidirectional causality between physiological and psychological (cognitive) systems has been described as follows: "it is impossible to make a clean *surgical* intervention in one system without its spreading to another system. All systems work together in much the same way as do the heart and lungs" (Beck, 1987b). As in the etiology of depression, cognition is assigned neither a "temporally primal" nor an exclusive "causal" role in the etiology of panic disorder (see also Beck, 1984a; White, 1990). Nevertheless, the cognitive component is theorized to be a necessary part of panic.

At what point within the "vicious panic cycle," conceptualized as a multiplicity of interacting physiological sensations and cognitive misinterpretations, does panic begin? To answer this question, we would need to define panic threshold intensity levels of various cognitive, affective, behavioral, and physiological symptoms of panic. In addition to this, there are concerns that since misinterpretations can be either conscious or unconscious, evidence to refute *temporal* primacy of catastrophic interpretations may be difficult to obtain (see McNally, 1990, p. 407). (McNally [1990, p. 407] has also suggested that "catastrophic misinterpretation" needs to be defined by measures that are empirically distinct from measures of panic itself. Though this philosophical point is beyond the scope of the present chapter, see R. S. Lazarus and Folkman, 1986, for a discussion of the issue of circularity in cognitive theories; criteria for avoiding circularity; and ways in which particular kinds of "circular" theories have proven to be of great value in discovering hitherto overlooked properties of a given phenomenon.)

Finally, the notion of "catastrophic" faulty attribution as the critical phenomenon in panic attacks is derived from contextually situated, complex clinical judgments. As such, the concept itself is causally complex rather than simple. Determining that a situation or stimulus is being misinterpreted as "catastrophic" requires the following: (1) an objective measure of the actual threat, if any; (2) a measure of the level of threat attached to the situation or stimulus by the panic patient; and (3) agreement on the magnitude of discrepancy between the objective and subjective threat measures that is necessary to define "catastrophic." Of course, as noted by Seligman (1988) and McNally (1990), this point does not negate the necessity for researchers to develop adequate measures of the construct. Rather, it emphasizes the complexity of the variables that must be taken into account in constructing the required measurements.

## TOWARD A UNIFIED PSYCHOLOGICAL THEORY OF PANIC DISORDER

Cognitive theory postulates relationships among several interacting levels (or "systems") of analysis (Beck, 1984b, 1985a). According to theoretical axiom 3 in Chapter 1, the influences between cognitive systems and other systems are bidirectional. Cognitive theory never was founded on the assumption of differences in processes or mechanisms of action between behavioral and cognitive therapies; instead, the conceptual overlap between cognitive therapy and behavior therapy has been emphasized (Beck, 1970a). From both perspectives, cognitive processes are theorized to be central to the conduct of effective therapy. In this regard, cognitive theory would appear to be a parsimonious perspective, since it provides a theoretical explanation to account for the efficacy of (or therapeutic processes underlying) the various models (see Beck, 1984b).

The experimental findings from human cognition and conditioning studies on which extrapolation to clinical disorder rests now suggest that the nature of conditioning is intricately connected to cognitive processes. Hence, it is not clear that distinct experimental predictions based on a "conditioning" model that excludes information or cognitive processing can now be made. Indeed, Rapee (1991a, p. 194) has argued that at a process level, conditioning theories can be conceptualized as a subset of cognitive theories. Our unified model itself would suggest this to be the case.

# CHAPTER SEVEN

# Schizophrenia and Other Psychotic Disorders

As noted in Chapter 5, Coyne (1994) has suggested that the domain of integrative psychotherapy must shrink if cognitive theory is appropriated as an integrative paradigm. However, this chapter provides further evidence that this view is not grounded in a complete understanding of the scope of cognitive theory. For example, in cognitive therapy, variables such as emotions and complex interpersonal processes within (and outside) the therapy session are not ignored or "reduced" to cognition. Cognitive therapists cover the same issues as interpersonal therapists do, but they explicitly attempt to produce cognitive change. Indeed, most of our discussions with patients revolve around interpersonal issues (Beck & Hollon, 1993, p. 91), and special attention has always been given to the interpersonal relationship between client and therapist (Beck et al., 1979, Ch. 3).

In this chapter, we devote attention to the theory, assessment, and treatment of schizophrenia and other psychotic disorders—among the most recent areas of exploration for the application of cognitive therapy (Chadwick & Birchwood,

1996).[1] These disabling, chronic disorders pose special challenges to the cognitive therapist, and their degree of complexity necessitates a particularly unified or "integrative" approach to therapy. Issues covered include the following: (1) the importance of idiographic assessment; (2) an example of incorporating basic research into the clinical practice of cognitive therapy; (3) distancing or perspective taking; (4) the need to focus on both cognitive content (e.g., delusional beliefs) and cognitive processing errors (cognitive distortions); (5) the importance of attention to interpersonal relationships with significant others outside treatment, as well as to the therapeutic alliance; (6) the focus on emotions; (7) expressed emotion and interpersonal stress; (8) treatment of negative self-concept; and (9) ecological validity. In addition, we present a brief review of the empirical status of cognitive treatments for psychotic disorders.

## IDIOGRAPHIC ASSESSMENT

There is an intriguing simplicity to the adaptation of cognitive therapy to treat schizophrenia and other psychotic disorders. Traditional cognitive therapy has been designed to treat disordered cognitive content (such as negativity) and disordered cognitive processes (such as dichotomous thinking). This approach has been successful in the treatment of disorders that have not historically been viewed as essentially cognitive in nature (Dobson, 1989; Hollon et al., 1992; Robins & Hayes, 1993). Therefore, the possibility of applying cognitive therapy to treat schizophrenia and other disorders that involve delusional beliefs (which are clearly significant disturbances of cognition) may appear self-evident.

---

[1]Portions of this chapter are adapted from Alford and Beck (1994) and Alford and Correia (1994). Copyright 1994 by Elsevier Science Ltd. and by the Association for Advancement of Behavior Therapy, respectively. Adapted by permission.

Concurrent pharmacotherapy and other adjunctive treatments are usually necessary in the treatment of psychotic disorders. Pharmacological, psychological, and social/interpersonal interventions all play a role in treatment of these complex disorders. Cognitive therapists routinely utilize pharmacological treatments, and employ cognitive therapy to enhance compliance, in addition to focusing on the cognitive aspects of social, interpersonal, and psychological factors (e.g., Fritze, Forthner, Schmitt, & Thaler, 1988; Perris, 1989).

Given the highly idiosyncratic nature of delusional beliefs and other symptoms, clinical assessment of the psychotic patient is necessarily individualized rather than nomothetic. However, standard cognitive therapy interview strategies can be employed successfully, with greater attention given to establishing and maintaining the interpersonal relationship (as described below). For theoretical reasons articulated below, assessment (and treatment) of psychotic disorders is similar to the assessment (and treatment) of personality disorders (see Beck et al., 1990).

In the beginning stages of assessment, the psychotic patient not only may be relatively unaware of the frequency of his or her delusional thoughts, but also may be unaware that the thoughts are abnormal. During the initial interview, the therapist maintains a neutral stance and communicates no surprise or overly skeptical reactions to the delusional material. A list of relevant beliefs is obtained, and the therapist suggests that the patient keep a daily log to record the frequency of specific thoughts that represent the beliefs. The exact mechanics of such recordings is adapted to what each patient considers feasible. For example, hospitalized inpatients may be able to record frequency of thoughts as they occur throughout the day, but an employed outpatient may find such a procedure interruptive of daily activities. Also, inpatients who suffer from chronic schizophrenia are often unable to record their own thoughts, because of such factors as limited intelligence, writing skills, and/or motivation. Cognitive therapists must then utilize therapist-administered time-sampled assessment (e.g., approaching an inpatient four times per day and assessing various clinical dimensions).

The most central important variable to be assessed in patients with delusions is the degree to which they may hold a specific delusional beliefs to be valid. This can be assessed by means of a subjective rating scale with a range from 0% to 100%. An interesting finding by Hole et al., (1979) was that the interviewing process itself, during which conviction ratings were determined, often decreased such ratings. This was the case even though the interviewers at this stage were merely interested in the phenomenology of the delusional beliefs, rather than in changing such beliefs.

The most likely explanation for the Hole et al. (1979) findings is that the act of systematically obtaining conviction ratings activates metacognitive processing, which results in a reduction of conviction. "Metacognition" means knowledge of the cognitive enterprise itself, including both cognitive content and processing activities (see Flavell, 1984; Johnson & White, 1971). Socratic questioning assesses conviction of psychopathological beliefs and explores with the patient the nature of the evidence necessary to evaluate such beliefs properly. Therefore, assessment and treatment activities are interrelated.

## INCORPORATING BASIC RESEARCH: THE EXAMPLE OF PSYCHOLOGICAL REACTANCE

Cognitive theory continues to incorporate principles derived from basic psychological research on processes such as development, cognition, and social interaction (cf. Rust, 1990). Principles regarding psychological reactance may be especially relevant to the clinical treatment of delusions (J. W. Brehm, 1966; S. S. Brehm, 1976). "Psychological reactance" is roughly identical to the phenomena the psychoanalytic theorists term "resistance" and the behaviorists "countercontrol." In the present context, reactance is shown in the special difficulties that cognitive therapists encounter as they assist psychotic patients in correcting their delusional beliefs. Cognitive therapy of schizophrenia and other psychotic disorders frequently results in a high rate of refusal and early treatment termination (e.g., Tarrier et al., 1993).

The DSM-IV criteria for paranoid schizophrenia (American Psychiatric Association, 1994, p. 287) include preoccupation with delusions (which are generally persecutory and/or grandiose), and anger and argumentativeness are associated features. Thus, this particular form of schizophrenia may contain within itself elements that increase reactance to treatment interventions. However, S. S. Brehm's (1976) theory predicts that changing delusional beliefs may be expected to create maximum reactance, even without a possible predisposition to "resist" treatment on the part of certain delusional patients. Determinants of magnitude of reactance include (1) the importance of the specific freedom that is being threatened (e.g., the freedom to have one's own thoughts, even if they are delusional), and (2) the magnitude of the threat (e.g., having to give up delusional beliefs entirely, rather than only partially changing them). Accordingly, changing such beliefs may generally be predicted to create high levels of reactance. Such private cognitive behaviors are important to the patient, and the therapist is asking that the patient give them up entirely.

Clinical studies that have reported successful modification of delusional beliefs have typically employed strategies that would be expected to minimize reactance. Chadwick and Lowe (1990) emphasize how their "reality-testing" procedure gives special attention to the collaborative approach: "In such cases the client and researcher collaborated to devise a simple test of the belief (see Hole, Rush, & Beck, 1979). . . . . An important principle behind the reality testing was that the client agreed in advance that the chosen task was a genuine test of the belief" (p. 227). This would be expected to reduce reactance by enhancing the patients' freedom to "have their own thoughts" (S. S. Brehm, 1976). Cognitive therapists emphasize that reason and observed evidence (rather than a therapist's opinion) should determine whether a belief is held or relinquished.

## DISTANCING OR PERSPECTIVE TAKING

The interrelated processes of identifying, monitoring, and evaluating thoughts and beliefs are applied directly to the treatment of psychotic symptoms. These standard cognitive therapy techniques facilitate distancing from thoughts. "Distancing" refers to the ability to view one's own thoughts (or beliefs) as constructions of "reality" rather than as reality itself. In one technique, a patient may be asked whether others seem to agree or disagree with the patient's views regarding delusional material. The patient can be led through guided discovery to recognize a discrepancy between his or her own perspective and that of others. Then the therapist conducts a dialogue with the patient to discuss how best to account for the difference. Therapist and patient focus directly on evaluating the evidence upon which the belief is based (as in Alford, 1986; Beck, 1952; Himadi et al., 1993; Kingdon & Turkington, 1991b; Tarrier, 1992). When psychotic patients are encouraged to take the perspective of other people temporarily, they are better able to distance themselves from their abnormal beliefs. This is consistent with the finding by Harrow and Miller (1980) that "[perspective-taking impairment] in schizophrenics is selective, involving difficulty in maintaining perspective on their own behavior, with better perspective when assessing others' behavior" (p. 717). Of course, this approach may be useful not only for those with schizophrenia, but also for those with other disorders, and for people engaging in normal, everyday problem solving as well.

Following the principle of using graded task assignments, cognitive therapists initially target those beliefs with the lowest conviction ratings. Such beliefs may be expected to be less resistant to treatment; thus, targeting them first increases the chances for establishing a nonthreatening therapeutic relationship. Since directly *challenging* beliefs has been associated with negative reactions on the part of some delusional patients (see Greenwood, 1983; Milton, Patwa, & Hafner, 1978; Wincze et al., 1972), the alternative strategy is to take a Socratic stance to collaboratively *test* beliefs. As an example, a therapist might ask a patient, "Do others seem to agree with you regarding [delusion]?" If the patient answers, "No," then the therapist might ask, "How do we account for that?" This would be followed by a dialogue to consider the evidence upon which the belief is based.

This approach avoids having the therapist appear to have all the answers. Experiments are devised as direct tests of the belief. Instead of "taking the therapist's word," the therapist and patient collaborate to devise a test of the belief that is agreeable to both of them (see Chadwick & Lowe, 1990).

This strategy was used in a case reported by Tarrier (1992). A patient, Tom, believed he must shout back at hallucinated voices in order to avoid being physically attacked. Tarrier (1992) described the test and outcome as follows:

> If the voices were real and Tom's belief true then a failure to argue should result in an attack. If the therapist's view that the voices were a symptom of his illness was true then no attack should occur. . . . When Tom was seen again 3 days later . . . [he] agreed that he had not been attacked and although his belief in the voices being real was still strong, he felt greatly relieved and much less concerned for his own safety. (p. 163)

## COGNITIVE CONTENT AND COGNITIVE PROCESSING

A distinction can be made between treatment of cognitive content and cognitive processes. For example, Spaulding, Storms, Goodrich, and Sullivan (1986) delineate "process-oriented" and "content-oriented" subcategories of cognitive interventions. Adams, Malatesta, Brantley, and Turkat (1981, pp. 460, 463) likewise write:

> The goal of this approach is remediation of deficits in cognitive processes rather than changing supposedly distorted cognitions (i.e., thoughts, attitudes, beliefs), which is typically the goal of cognitive behavior therapy. . . . Behavioral approaches to modify cognitive processes should not be confused with cognitive behavior therapy. The latter approach is concerned with modifying specific cognitions or distorted attitudes and beliefs about oneself or the environment. Disorders of cognitive processes such as schizophrenia require intervention directed at the processes themselves and not at the specific cognitions.

Cognitive theory posits interrelated constructs to explain the nature of dysfunctional cognitive processing and content in the various psychopathological conditions. The principle of cognitive content specificity (axiom 4, Chapter 1) predicts specific cognitive content in the various disorders. For example, hopelessness (negative view of the future) is theoretically implicated in depression; threat themes are related to anxiety; and concepts of mistreatment or abuse by others are related to anger control disorders. No such specificity has been theorized for the various kinds of cognitive processing errors, with the possible exception of a link between dichotomous thinking and borderline personality disorder (Beck et al., 1990, p. 187).

A defining characteristic of cognitive therapy is the correction of specific cognitive distortions in the various forms of psychopathology (Beck, 1976). Clearly, patients with schizophrenia and other psychotic disorders suffer from many of the classic cognitive distortions that have been the focus of cognitive therapy for well over 30 years now(Beck, 1991b). We find patient reports replete with examples of this point. In regard to personalization, for instance, patient Mary McGrath (quoted in Hatfield, 1989, p. 1142) provides this description of her experience: "I am frightened too when every whisper, every laugh is about me." On dichotomous thinking, Nona Borgeson (also quoted in Hatfield, 1989, p. 1142) writes: "Where weighing the odds of probability ends, schizophrenia begins, and paranoia runs rampant. . . . [A patient's world becomes one of polarities—black or white, love or hate, ecstasy or suicidal inclinations, mortal fear or indestructibility."

The cognitive therapist working with a psychotic patient focuses on changing both disordered cognitive processing and maladaptive cognitive content. Treatment of the specific distortions in cognitive processing (e.g., personalization, arbitrary inference, dichotomous thinking, and selective abstraction) is as important as is the treatment of maladaptive cognitive content. To take an example, consider the case of Daniel. Daniel believed that various people had been "spying" on him for several years (cognitive content). The processing errors of personalization and arbitrary inference (cognitive distortions) were also observed. Daniel had recently been involved in an automobile accident, and these paranoid beliefs and processing errors were prominent in his account of this event. In the initial interview, the following discussion took place:

Patient: These people have been after me for years now. This is nothing new for me.

Therapist: The same people who followed you when you drove off into the cornfield have been after you for years?

Patient: Yes. But they drove away when they saw my car run off the road. They never actually confront me.

Therapist: Let's review how they followed you this most recent time when you had the accident in your car, OK?

Patient: OK.

Therapist: When did the "following" begin?

Patient: When I left my house to go to the convenience store.

Therapist: Tell me about *how* that happened. [Note: *"How"* focuses on process.]

Patient: I went to the first stop sign and there they were. Every time I turned, they turned. So I decided to lose them and drove out of town. They followed me, as I knew they would.

Therapist: Now, *how* did you know they were following you?

Patient: They turned every time I did.

Therapist: Are there other possibilities as to why they might have turned every time you did?

Patient: No. At first I thought that, but then, when they followed me out of town, I knew *they* were following me.

Therapist: Were there any other people going out of town at the same time you were, besides the people you thought were following you?

Patient: (*Pause*) Yes. But when I speeded up, they speeded up. At one point, we were going over 110 miles an hour! They were laughing and pointing at me. Then I knew who they were.

In the example above, the processing errors of personalization and arbitrary inference were related to a specific belief (content): "These people have been after me for years." The patient in this case correctly observed the "fact" that he was being followed, but the interpretation or meaning of his being followed was incorrect; in other words, cognitive distortion/processing errors were present. To treat these, the therapist encouraged Daniel in subsequent sessions to consider how he had made inferences ("guesses") without sufficient supporting evidence.

Information from the police officers who investigated the accident—information that Daniel had initially rejected as untrue—was presented in this discussion. Several teenagers admitted they had indeed been following him, but had not done so until he himself began to increase his speed. He noticed them and thought he was being followed. Alternative interpretations regarding the intentions of those persons following the patient were discussed, and the (arbitrary) inferences regarding the high-speed chase were considered. The teens had simply thought, "This guy wants to race!"

## THE INTERPERSONAL CONTEXT

In cognitive therapy, the interpersonal context of psychiatric disorder is given careful attention. For example, faulty family interactions are a frequent source of stress for patients with schizophrenia. It is well documented that family interactions are involved in the generation of stress, and that stress is implicated in the activation of schizophrenic symptoms (Clements & Turpin, 1992; Hatfield, 1989; Zubin & Spring, 1977). Schizophrenic patients experience greater stress reactions for several reasons, including their tendency to underappraise their internal resources (minimization) (Hatfield, 1989; Wasylenki, 1992).

Employing the cognitive technique of graded task assignments, Allen and Bass (1992) used (1) low-expectancy communications and (2) graded practice to treat two patients with schizophrenia. Such an approach places minimal demands on cognitive resources (see Heinssen & Victor, 1994; McGlashan, Heinssen, & Fenton, 1989). Caseworkers explicitly sympathized with the patients and "normalized" their stressful experiences. Individualized graded-practice programs were designed to facilitate success at each step in approaching problem situations. Patients improved in measures of "fight and flight" behaviors and positive symptoms (hallucinations, incoherent speech, and delusions). Limitations of this study, however, included lack of multiple baselines, no follow-up, a poorly formulated diathesis–stress framework, and no attention to therapeutic process to confirm that the results were specifically attributable to the therapy (Allen & Bass, 1992).

Kingdon and Turkington (1991b) correctly note the importance of treating the dysfunctional interpersonal relationships between schizophrenic patients and members of their families. They note that family members catastrophize psychotic symptoms as much as patients do, and describe how this leads to criticism and stress within these families. To correct this, Kingdon and Turkington (1991b) explore the use of "normalizing" conceptualizations of psychotic symptoms. Articulation of the continuum between culturally acceptable beliefs and delusional beliefs serves a destigmatizing function for patients and their families. Psychopathology may be further normalized by showing the role of stress in onset of symptoms. Concurrently, the cognitive distortions are treated, "particularly personalization (taking things personally), selective abstraction (getting things out of context) and arbitrary inference (jumping to conclusions)" (p. 208). They report that among 64 consecutive patients who were treated in this manner, there was little need for medication, and only a minimum of hospitalization was necessary.

A four-part intervention—education about schizophrenia; stress management; setting goals; and stress inoculation—was tested by Barrowclough and Tarrier (1987). The patient was a 29-year-old male who lived with his parents. Both parents attended all sessions. At the outset of treatment, there had been three previous hospitalizations, and the time between relapses had shortened. Treatment appeared to reduce relapse rate, improve social functioning, and significantly reduce measures of stressors ("expressed emotion," discussed later in this chapter) within the family.

## THE FOCUS ON EMOTIONS

One of the most common misconceptions about cognitive therapy is that it does not focus on emotional experiences and expressions in clinical treatment (Gluhoski, 1994; Weishaar, 1993). However, to facilitate understanding of the phenomenological perspective of the delusional patient, the cognitive therapist must closely attend to the emotions associated with delusional thoughts and beliefs (Alford & Beck, 1994). In some cases, knowing the patient's emotional state during the activation of specific beliefs may assist in understanding the maintenance of such beliefs. In other cases, successful treatment of delusional beliefs may be facilitated by attending to the more positive feelings associated with alternative explanations of events that up to now have been misinterpreted in negative delusional terms. If the consequent affect shift is substantial and positive, the patient will be more strongly motivated to consider evidence incongruent with the maladaptive belief. Thus, attention to associated emotions is crucial in the cognitive therapy of delusional ideation. Cognitive therapists identify and explore feelings associated with the various presenting delusional beliefs, as well as feelings about the possibility that the delusions are incorrect.

The interpersonal framework of cognitive therapy dictates that specific techniques (Socratic dialogue, normalizing rationale, belief-testing experiments, reattribution, etc.) be utilized to accomplish therapeutic goals established *within the context of a collaborative relationship with the patient*. This component of cognitive therapy is extremely important to the success of cognitive therapy of schizophrenia and delusional beliefs (Alford & Beck, 1994). A "cognitive technique" does not exist apart from the context of the collaborative relationship within which cognitive therapy takes place; the strategies used in therapy are jointly developed and implemented.

The interpersonal relationship in cognitive therapy is of course highly structured. Factors to be discussed and agreed upon include expectations for therapy, an agenda for each session, the nature of the patient's problems, and goals for treatment. Most important are discussion and agreement about the specific rationales for the various techniques used during therapy. As elaborated in Chapter 1, techniques used in cognitive therapy are employed *with*, not applied to, the patient.

In addition to the development of techniques to test beliefs, cognitive therapy of psychotic disorders focuses on the patient's struggle to come to terms with his or her condition (as in the case of Jack, below). If the patient is to accomplish this, a greater focus on the interpersonal relationship is required than in many other disorders.

In an early study of a patient with chronic schizophrenia, Beck (1952) described his own role as predominantly supportive and educative: "I was relatively nondirective in allowing him to bring up whatever he felt was important" (p. 307). Therapy also included techniques such as identifying interconnections among external stresses, emotions, and symptoms (delusional beliefs). The patient's delusional belief was that 50 different customers of his father's small retail store (where the patient worked) were FBI agents. Therapy focused on reducing delusions regarding these specific customers. After 30 sessions over 8 months, the following was reported: "On the occasions when he would start to suspect that one of his customers was an agent he would reason [himself] out of it. He reported that he was able to narrow down the original group of fifty to two or three possibilities and that he felt he would soon be able to eliminate them completely" (Beck, 1952, p. 310). Although the patient was assisted in identifying the original experiences that had preceded his delusional beliefs and in systematically testing his conclusions, the interpersonal focus was deemed most essential to treatment. Beck wrote: "The major force in the therapeutic process appears to have been the emotional experience between patient and therapist" (1952, p. 311).

Hole et al. (1979) likewise emphasized the relatively nondirective aspects of cognitive treatment of delusions. Interviews of eight delusional patients were structured in a nonconfrontational manner, and were designed to identify the phenomenology of each belief: "[The interviewer] tried to engage the patient in a joint exploration of certain questions: Did the belief rest on current experience? How did he [sic] process information inconsistent with the belief? If there was some change in any aspect of the belief, how did the patient account for the change?" (Hole et al., 1979, p. 314).

The view others take of a patient's delusional beliefs will determine their behavior toward him or her. For example, a patient may believe that hallucinated voices can be controlled only by verbal counterattacks (Tarrier, 1992). Family members who fail to understand the reason for such outbursts may think that such behavior is directed toward themselves (personalization). They may then become angry at the patient and increase the patient's stress. The therapist must first understand the patient's behavior from the patient's point of view, and then bring family members into therapy to inform them of the meaning of such behavior. Concurrently, the patient is led to reconsider the need for the verbally aggressive responses to the hallucinated voices, as the interpersonal stress caused by family members' counterattacks toward the patient is attenuated. As negative interactions decrease, the cognitive resources available to the patient for his or her own personal therapy (as opposed to coping with the interpersonal stressors) will increase.

In the manner described above, cognitive therapy treats interpersonal problems so as to reduce the stressors implicated in the onset and maintenance of psychotic symptoms. Reattributing delusions as continuous with normal experiences (e.g., identifying how stress increases symptoms) teaches patients' families to view the symptoms and the patients as less bizarre. This facilitates improvement in the patients' poor self-concept, resulting in still further improvement. Moreover, as discussed below, when those within a delusional patient's interpersonal network understand the symptoms to be caused by a psychological disorder, fewer expressions of blame or other stress-inducing communications are directed to the patient.

## EXPRESSED EMOTION AND INTERPERSONAL STRESS

In the standard practice of cognitive therapy, cognitive therapists do not exclude significant others from therapy sessions when interpersonal conflicts relate to a patient's complaints. The use of interpersonal cognitive strategies in work with psychotic patients relates to studies on "expressed emotion" (EE) (Alford & Beck, 1994). Because delusional beliefs occur in an interpersonal context, the cognitive therapist addresses interpersonal factors in treatment (cf. Beck, 1988b). Family therapy is prescribed for such patients. In families rated high in EE, schizophrenia relapse rates have been shown to decrease after family interventions, as compared to control and routine treatments (Barrowclough & Tarrier, 1992).

The concept of EE has recently been subjected to behavioral (but not cognitive) assessment (Halford, 1991). A thorough assessment of EE would explore the patient's and family members' thoughts and underlying beliefs. A possible sequence for assessment might be the following: Beliefs lead to automatic thoughts, which lead in turn to EE.

Family members typically have contrasting beliefs about numerous issues related to a psychotic patient. A mother may believe that "My son has a mental disorder," and "I'm responsible for supporting him and helping him overcome the delusions." The father may believe that "My son has a motivation problem," and "He could get better if he tried harder." Consequently, the mother may be inclined to interpret a situation, such as the son's failing to keep his bedroom in order, as follows: "Sick children should not be expected to be neat and orderly." The father's opposing belief (that the schizo-phrenic son lacks motivation) may lead him to attach an opposite meaning to the same event: "This boy should be disciplined." Faulty interpersonal relationships will probably follow.

The existence of incompatible beliefs is manifested when family interactions among the mother, father, and son activate automatic thoughts regarding a specific event. The involuntary thoughts and associated emotions generated in a specific situation or interaction will be related to the dysfunctional beliefs. To continue with the example above, if the father finds the son's bedroom to be disorderly, his beliefs will be activated and may generate successively the following possible thoughts and associated emotions: "He is getting worse because I am too weak to discipline him" (sadness); "It's his fault—he could get better" (anger); "I'd better demand that he do better or he will really get crazy" (fear). The mother's initial interpretation of the son's bedroom in disarray will likewise be schema-driven. Her own negative automatic thoughts and associated emotions may include these: "I've failed" (sadness); "My husband is going to be angry" (fear); "He [her husband] is too strict and puts too many demands on our child" (anger). Thus, the differing perspectives are likely to lead to arguments.

Expression of these emotions is lawfully related to the respective thoughts and underlying beliefs regarding specific interpersonal events within the family. The emotional response generated will depend upon the underlying meanings associated with the topographical thoughts. The principle of cognitive content specificity applies to both private emotion and EE (see R. S. Lazarus, 1991a, 1991c). The assessment or determination of the specific meanings associated with a given thought allows us to predict the concomitant emotional reaction.

As family members interact (as in the example given above), automatic thoughts and associated emotions become public. In this manner, the psychotic patient's environment becomes more stressful as he or she tries to understand the meaning of the others' arguments. In the example above, the son himself is likely to become involved in the conflict between the mother and father, and to bring his own maladaptive beliefs into the interactions. If the son believes that "I'm causing all the problems," his self-esteem is likely to suffer.

To summarize, EE is theorized to be derived from specific automatic thoughts, which in turn are derived from idiosyncratic maladaptive schemas. The various emotional responses within a family are inextricably linked to specific cognitive processes (R. S. Lazarus, 1991a), disorders of which (both in content and in processing) have been implicated in the various clinical syndromes (Beck, 1991b). Future research programs should seek to uncover the precise mechanisms linking EE to higher relapse in schizophrenia (as in Barrowclough & Tarrier, 1992) by conducting idiographic cognitive assessment of EE, as suggested above.

## THE FOCUS ON SELF-CONCEPT

Another common misconception regarding cognitive therapy is that it does not focus on the self-concept and personality in clinical treatment (Gluhoski, 1994; Weishaar, 1993). As described in Alford and Beck (1994), the treatment of delusional patients involves special problems in developing a working therapeutic relationship. Such patients typically experience severe problems in relating to others, which are secondary to their extremely distorted view of themselves, the world, and other people. Especially relevant is the presence of a negative self-concept (see Bentall, Kinderman, & Kaney, 1994). Consider the following case of Jack.

In the initial session, Jack described a long history of obviously paranoid beliefs, which had created significant problems in his adjustment to both his past and present environments. A review of this patient's history showed that he had dropped out of medical school, largely because of a belief that professors were "talking about" him and were (in his words) "after me—trying to get something on me." At the time Jack sought treatment, he was experiencing similar cognitions, which were threatening his current employment.

Jack believed the same people who had earlier been "after" him had now located him, even though he had intentionally moved hundreds of miles from his previous location. He now believed that they were "monitoring my every move," and that several federal agencies were involved. He attributed a personalized meaning to specific billboards that had recently been erected; he thought they were intended to communicate to him, "You have been found."

One central problem in attempting to establish a collaborative relationship with Jack was his initial *apparent* 100% conviction that these various agencies and persons were indeed plotting against him. (Actually, as shown below, he had grave and quite disturbing doubts regarding the correctness of these paranoid beliefs.) He initially described his presenting problem thus: "I need someone to help me cope with the stress caused by these people."

To pose an alternative, mutually agreeable agenda, the therapist suggested the goal of first evaluating the evidence that there was in fact such a threat; if such a threat was found, then the therapist and patient would jointly explore ways to handle the persons responsible for the alleged harassment. At that point, the following conversation took place:

Therapist: How would you feel about adding that [an exploration of the beliefs] as an agenda item or goal for our collaborative efforts?

Patient: I don't know . . . I would not want to find that it was all me.

Therapist: What do you mean?

Patient: I think that would be worse than finding out that there is a conspiracy.

Therapist: It would seem to me that you would not really want all those agencies and people after you. Wouldn't that be a bigger problem?

Patient: Not really. I would not want to find out I've been the cause of all this.

Therapist: How would you feel if you did find that to be the case?

Patient: (*Hesitating; tears in eyes*) I would be afraid.

Therapist: Of what?

Patient: It would mean that I've *really* got a problem.

It was obvious that therapy should not proceed directly to the collaborative development of techniques to test Jack's beliefs. Instead, the focus shifted to analysis and compassionate understanding of this patient's struggle to come to terms with his condition. Jack's recognition of the discrepancy between his beliefs and reality indicated the nascent activation of metacognitive processing, or distancing from his thoughts. Wouldn't anyone be disconcerted to recognize the meaning one attached to events to be so markedly unrealistic? The most critical clinical strategy with patients who experience delusional beliefs is to deal constructively with the issue of the existence of delusions as such, and with the means the patients attach to the presence of such experiences.

A patient who is cognizant of holding markedly abnormal ideas is at risk of suffering loss of self-esteem (and increased anxiety) when such ideas are discussed during treatment. Consequently, the cognitive therapist must be especially sensitive to avoid threats to the patient's self-esteem (see Dingman & McGlashan, 1989; Lyon, Kaney, & Bentall, 1994), and must apply standard cognitive therapy to restructure the negative self-concept.

## ECOLOGICAL VALIDITY

Spaulding et al. (1986) and Spaulding, Garbin, and Crinean (1989) have recently reviewed the status of clinical psychological treatment of schizophrenia. Among the important issues reviewed is the question of whether "experimental psychopathology" findings can be directly applied to the clinical treatment of schizophrenia (see also Green, 1993).

Spaulding et al. (1986) note that patients with schizophrenia have been shown in countless studies to have deficits in basic psychological functions (e.g., attention, memory, perception, and concept formation). Many such deficits have been found amenable to correction by specific techniques (see Riskind, 1991). In describing a technique designed to teach "concept modulation" to a 23-year-old patient with schizophrenia, Spaulding et al. (1986) write:

> The nature of the deficit was hypothesized to be a tendency to schematize a situation rapidly, and then perseverate with that schematization despite changes in the situation. [Note: The cognitive therapy term for this particular distortion, or processing error, is "overgeneralization."] . . . An exercise was designed to increase his ability to reconceptualize a social situation rapidly, and reject his stereotype. For 10 therapy sessions, the patient was asked to generate alternative schematizations, first to inkblots and then to Thematic Apperception Test (TAT) cards. That is, he was instructed to generate as many different percepts (to the inkblots) or stories (to the TAT cards) as he could to a single stimulus. (p. 571)

This procedure was used along with counseling, which focused on the importance of conceptual flexibility in social situations. The combined treatment seemed to work (Spaulding et al., 1986).

Numerous studies have clearly shown that schizophrenic and other psychotic patients have specific deficits such as those assessed by Spaulding et al. (1986): "simple reaction time, backward masking, span of apprehension, distraction effects on the reaction time task, redundancy-associated effects on the reaction time task, vigilance, and size estimation" (p. 571). However, such deficits are contextually situated within complex social environments. Harrow and Miller (1980) found impaired "perspective taking," defined as follows: "*Perspective*, in the sense we have used it, refers to the ability to recognize, in global fashion and in terms of broad consensual standards, which particular verbalizations and behavior are appropriate for a particular situation" (p. 717; emphasis in original). Similarly, J. D. Cohen, Servan-Schreiber, Targ, and Spiegel (1992) emphasize a higher-level cognitive function, disordered "context processing," to account for schizophrenic behavior. Thus, cognitive disorders in schizophrenia are dysfunctional or maladaptive in specific environmental contexts, and consequently in unique or personal ways.

Cognitive deficits such as simple reaction time may be studied experimentally. And discrete deficits, identified independently of the natural environmental context, may properly be a focus of cognitive rehabilitation efforts. Yet the patient described by Spaulding et al. (1986) showed "belligerent behavior and hostile demeanor" (p. 571), which had precluded his admission to a residential psychosocial treatment program. The generation of alternative schematizations to the inkblots and TAT does not constitute as direct an approach as possible alternatives, such as treating the patient's overgeneralization error, which was associated with maladaptive anger in specific natural contexts. This example is relevant to the recent convergence of attention on the importance of contextual variables among clinical behaviorists (Biglan, Glasgow, & Singer, 1990; Jacobson, 1992). The emphasis on context concerns whether treatments produce changes that will persist across situations (Baer, Wolf, & Risley, 1987).

Further research is needed to determine when an intervention directed at natural environments (see, e.g., Alford & Jaremko, 1990), as opposed to one directed at basic levels of cognitive dysfunction, may result in clinically significant differential outcomes and relapse prevention. In standard cognitive therapy, the question of whether or not remediation of basic cognitive deficits generalize to complex social environments does not arise. Through cognitive therapy homework experiments, cognitive remediation itself takes place in the natural environment. Thus, ecological validity is assessed continually during treatment.

## EMPIRICAL STATUS OF COGNITIVE TREATMENTS: A REVIEW

Schizophrenic and other psychotic disorders are characterized by disturbances of both thought form (process) and content. Positive treatment outcomes in the cognitive clinical treatment of such chronic disorders are, of course, not always obtained. However, preliminary studies now suggest a special application for cognitive therapy in the treatment of these relatively intractable conditions (Alford & Beck, 1994; Alford & Correia, 1994; Morrison, 1994; Morrison, Haddock, & Tarrier, in press).

Clinical reports have long suggested the possibility of success with this patient population. For example, an early study of a chronic schizophrenic patient (reviewed above in "The Focus on Emotions") showed that the patient was eventually able to achieve some distance from his delusional productions (Beck, 1952). Kingdon and Turkington (1991a) describe this case (Beck, 1952) as the first to employ reasoning techniques in the treatment of delusional thinking and beliefs, and thus to suggest the experimental application of cognitive therapy to treat psychotic disorders.

The empirical status of cognitive therapy of schizophrenia and other psychotic disorders has recently been discussed elsewhere (Alford & Beck, 1994; Alford & Correia, 1994). Outcome studies, including both individual therapy approaches and combined approaches (family, individual, and stress reduction combinations), suggest the usefulness of cognitive approaches to psychotic symptoms. Several of these outcome studies are briefly reviewed here.

An early cognitive approach to schizophrenia was reported by Watts, Powell, and Austin (1973). The patients were three individuals whose schizophrenia included severe paranoid delusional beliefs. The experimenters conducted a preliminary interview and constructed a list of statements that reflected subjects' abnormal beliefs; 20 statements for the first patient, 23 for the second, and 40 for the third were identified. A 5-point scale was used to rate strength of belief in each statement, prior to and following the cognitive intervention. Four principles were applied in therapy:

1. The more strongly rated beliefs were treated first in order to minimize psychological reactance, or resistance. The experimenters made efforts to modify the more strongly held beliefs only after reduction of the weaker beliefs was achieved.

2. Patients were asked to *consider* alternative beliefs, rather than simply to accept the views of the experimenters.

3. Emphasis was placed on evaluating the evidence on which a belief was based, not simply on evaluating the belief itself.

4. Participants were taught to articulate arguments against their own beliefs.

Results showed that ratings of strength of belief in delusional statements were lowered following therapy ($p < .02$ for subject 1, $p < .001$ for subjects 2 and 3). Control treatments (relaxation and *in vivo* desensitization procedures) for subjects 2 and 3 did not change strength-of-belief ratings from pretest to posttest (Watts et al., 1973).

An investigation by Hole et al. (1979), mentioned earlier in this chapter, tested a relatively nondirective, collaborative cognitive approach to delusions. Interviews were nonconfrontational and focused on the patients' introspective experience. Eight inpatients with schizophrenic delusions (two women, six men) participated in the study; they were chosen randomly from the University of Pennsylvania psychiatric services. For each belief, each patient provided ratings of conviction (certainty about the delusional idea, from 0% to 100%) and pervasiveness (time the patient spent thinking about or seeking the delusional goal).

Outcome was mixed. Four patients with severe chronic schizophrenia showed no significant changes in pervasiveness (high) or conviction (high) ratings. However, one patient did "accommodate" or alter a delusional belief when he was presented with data inconsistent with the belief. Two patients markedly reduced their pervasiveness ratings, but not their conviction ratings. At the same time, they did show overall clinical improvement in pursuing nondelusional goals and social concerns upon discharge. Two patients markedly reduced both pervasiveness and conviction ratings.

Alford (1986) reported the outcome of a 22-year-old inpatient with chronic paranoid schizophrenia. The patient's problems included delusional beliefs (the presence of a "haggly old witch") and behavioral disruptions linked to these ideas. Cognitive treatment was conducted from two to three times weekly. Alternative interpretations of beliefs and hallucinatory experiences were developed collaboratively with the patient. An A-B-A-B design, with placebo control sessions during baseline phases, showed a decrease in the strength of delusional beliefs during treatment. Members of the nursing staff, who were uninformed regarding experimental phases, reduced neuroleptic medications during active treatment phases (Alford, 1986). Three months after treatment, the patient's acquired metacognitive skills (self-monitoring and critical evaluation of thoughts) and behavioral improvements had partially persisted.

Another study, by Chadwick and Lowe (1990), likewise evaluated the effectiveness of cognitive treatment of delusional beliefs. Six outpatients who had had chronic schizophrenia for 2 or more years, and who had had delusional ideas for over 8 years, met with a researcher who expressed a wish to discuss the patients' beliefs. No participant was told the purpose of the study. Ratings of conviction (as in Alford, 1986, and Hole et al., 1979), preoccupation, and anxiety associated with the delusional beliefs were made; the patients provided these ratings for each belief following each session throughout the study. Each patient met with a researcher for weekly 1-hour sessions throughout the study. Phase 1 used interviews to establish rapport and define beliefs. During phase 2 (baseline), information was obtained on the patient's view of evidence for each delusional belief. A "verbal challenge" was given during phase 3; that is, the experimenter suggested the belief to be "only one possible interpretation of events." The patient's beliefs were not said to be incorrect, but the patient was asked to compare the experimenter's interpretations with his or her own. To develop metacognitive skills, the manner in which initial beliefs determine future processing of evidence was presented. Beliefs were challenged in three stages: (1) Logical inconsistencies were noted; (2) alternative explanations were given; and (3) the researcher directly suggested the alternative explanations to be better, and "reality-testing" demonstrations were provided as needed. By the end of the experiment, five of the six patients had reduced their conviction ratings. Improvement without symptom substitution was observed on a brief symptom checklist and on the Beck Depression Inventory, and this improvement was maintained at a 6-month follow-up.

In summary, the studies conducted to date suggest that cognitive approaches may play an increasingly important role in the treatment and management of psychotic symptoms. Standard cognitive therapy treats both disordered cognitive content and faulty cognitive processing ("formal thought disorder"). Cognitive therapy with schizophrenic and other psychotic patients emphasizes the establishment of the therapeutic relationship and attends to emotions. Standard cognitive therapy restructures the negative self-concept and, through homework assignments, facilitates ecological validity. Additional refinements are expected from the results of research projects currently underway.

# Epilogue

A central thesis of this volume is that certain characteristics of cognitive therapy may allow it to serve as a unifying paradigm for understanding the proximal and distal origins of psychopathology and the mechanisms of effective psychotherapy. As a scientific system of psychotherapy, cognitive therapy is grounded in a comprehensive theory of psychopathology. Its theory is consistent with the specific techniques applied by cognitive therapists in clinical practice. Its theoretical axioms are related logically to one another, and the theory is internally consistent, parsimonious, testable, and broad in its scope of application. Moreover, cognitive therapy is based on a tenable theory of personality (Beck, 1996; Beck, et al., 1990). Empirical outcome research and other studies have been conducted to demonstrate its effectiveness.

The scope of cognitive therapy has expanded to include many disorders in addition to clinical depression (the original focus of cognitive therapy and research). The preceding chapters have provided examples of how the cognitive focus of treatment has evolved along with this expanded scope of application. Indeed, a dichotomous focus (e.g., techniques vs. the interpersonal relationship) has never been the approach of cognitive therapy (see Beck et al., 1979, Ch. 3); it would be especially ineffective in the clinical treatment of complex disorders, such as those that are now being treated by cognitive therapists. Treatment strategies have evolved and become more specialized over the years, and treatment of each disorder requires special areas of competence.

Cognitive therapy has been shown to integrate a number of dimensions that have historically divided the various schools of psychotherapy. For example, in Chapter 2, we have shown how cognitive therapy resolves the question of internal versus external (environmental) dimensions or causes of psychopathology; we have articulated how cognitive theory incorporates environmental feedback (final causal) explanations of behavior, in addition to the more traditional "mechanistic" (efficient causal) accounts. The theoretical framework of cognitive therapy provides for a focus on interpersonal issues, emotions, and self-concept. It attends to both cognitive content and cognitive processes. Significant others are included in therapy sessions, and the environmental context is taken into account as a causal factor in psychopathology. Standard cognitive therapy does not neglect the focus on the unconscious, but rather seeks to make unconscious cognitive content conscious. Contrary to common misperceptions, cognitive therapy attends to past experiences, to the relationship with the therapist, and to relationships with significant others outside the therapy context. Thus, cognitive therapy not only deals effectively with domains typically associated with interpersonal, behavioral, and psychodynamic psychotherapy; it provides a unifying theoretical framework within which the clinical techniques of other established, validated psychotherapeutic approaches may be properly incorporated. By assimilating proven techniques that are theoretically consistent with the cognitive perspective, cognitive therapy provides a coherent, evolving paradigm for clinical practice.

Since the primary level of analysis in cognitive therapy is that of personal consciousness or meaning assignment—

that is, the focus is on the *patient's* view of events—a collaborative approach to treatment is insured. The importance of interpersonal factors (the "therapeutic relationship") in the psychotherapy process is given a great deal of emphasis in cognitive therapy, particularly in the treatment of chronic disorders. This is relevant to cognitive theory as integrative therapy, given the role of the therapeutic relationship as a common factor across the various psychotherapy systems.

Chapter 4 of this volume provides a critical consideration of issues within the contemporary movement to provide a comprehensive or "integrative" approach to psychotherapy. We have concluded that cognitive therapy—typically thought of as a unidimensional, "pure-form" therapy—is itself a comprehensive scientific system of psychotherapy that meets many of the goals of the integrationists. It includes technically eclectic clinical procedures, but bases these on a consistent theoretical framework that has proven to be a testable and, consequently, an evolving paradigm for clinical practice.

Finally, the psychotherapy integration movement has at the very least contributed to our appreciation for diversity and competition within the fields of psychopathology and psychotherapy. The contemporary psychotherapy integration movement itself—in seeking to replace the established systems with "integrative" approaches—has resulted in new rivalries. However, there would appear to be an optimal balance between cooperation (integration) and competition among schools of thought. Indeed, some within the integrationist movement have suggested that "chaos" rather than unification now prevails as a result of competition among the various schools of eclectic and integrative psychotherapy (A. A. Lazarus & Messer, 1991, p. 144). The solution to such conflict would appear to be coherent theories that are testable, and that are tested—both by those who advance them and by independent investigators. As reflected in the dedication of the present volume, many of the theories that compete with cognitive conceptualizations have served to help insure the continued evolution of cognitive theory. Competing scientific theories, like scholarly critics and researchers of cognitive therapy, play a dialectical role in the continuing evaluation and refinement of clinical cognitive theory.

# References

Adams, H. E., Malatesta, V., Brantley, P. J., & Turkat, I. D. (1981). Modification of cognitive processes: A case study of schizophrenia. *Journal of Consulting and Clinical Psychology, 49,* 460–464.

Ainslie, G. (1975). Specious reward: A behavioral theory of impulsiveness and impulse control. *Psychological Bulletin, 82,* 463–496.

Alford, B. A. (1984). Clinical effects of increasing goal relevant positive verbalizations within a naturally occurring verbal community (Doctoral dissertation, University of Mississippi, 1984). *Dissertation Abstracts International, 45-05B,* 1578. (University Microfilms No. 84–15,690)

Alford, B. A. (1986). Behavioral treatment of schizophrenic delusions: A single-case experimental analysis. *Behavior Therapy, 17,* 637–644.

Alford, B. A. (1991). Integration of scientific criteria into the psychotherapy integration movement. *Journal of Behavior Therapy and Experimental Psychiatry, 22*(3), 211–216.

Alford, B. A. (1993a). Brief cognitive psychotherapy of panic disorder. In R. A. Wells & V. J. Gianetti (Eds.), *Casebook of the brief psychotherapies* (pp. 65–75). New York: Plenum Press.

Alford, B. A. (1993b). Contextualistic behaviorism, radical behaviorism, and cognitive therapy. *The Behavior Therapist, 16,* 201–203.

Alford, B. A. (1995). Introduction to the special issue: "Psychotherapy integration" and cognitive psychotherapy. *Journal of Cognitive Psychotherapy: An International Quarterly, 9*(3), 147–151.

Alford, B. A. (in press). Theories of psychotherapy versus integrative ideology: A reply to Castonguay and Goldfried. *Applied and Preventive Psychology.*

Alford, B. A., & Beck, A. T. (1994). Cognitive therapy of delusional beliefs. *Behaviour Research and Therapy, 32*(3), 369–380.

Alford, B. A., Beck, A. T., Freeman, A., & Wright, F. D. (1990). Brief focused cognitive therapy of panic disorder. *Psychotherapy, 27*(2), 230–234.

Alford, B. A., & Carr, S. M. (1992). Cognition and classical conditioning in panic disorder. *The Behavior Therapist, 15*(6), 143–147.

Alford, B. A., & Correia, C. J. (1994). Cognitive therapy of schizophrenia: Theory and empirical status. *Behavior Therapy, 25,* 17–33.

Alford, B. A., & Jaremko, M. E. (1990). Behavioral design of a positive verbal community: A preliminary experimental analysis. *Journal of Behavior Therapy and Experimental Psychiatry, 21,* 173–184.

Alford, B. A., Lester, J., Patel, R., Buchanan, J. P., & Giunta, L. (1995). Hopelessness predicts future depressive symptoms: A prospective analysis of cognitive vulnerability and cognitive content specificity. *Journal of Clinical Psychology, 51,* 331–339.

Alford, B. A., & Norcross, J. C. (1991). Cognitive therapy as integrative therapy. *Journal of Psychotherapy Integration, 1*(3), 175–190.

Alford, B. A., Richards, C., & Hanych, J. (1995). The causal status of private events. *The Behavior Therapist, 18,* 57–58.

Allen, H., & Bass, C. (1992). Coping tactics and the management of acutely distressed schizophrenic patients. *Behavioural Psychotherapy, 20,* 61–72.

American Board of Professional Psychology (ABPP). (1996). *Manual for oral examinations.* Columbia, MO: Author.

American Psychiatric Association. (1968). *Diagnostic and statistical manual of mental disorders* (2nd ed.). Washington, DC: Author.

American Psychiatric Association. (1994). *Diagnostic and statistical manual of mental disorders* (4th ed.). Washington, DC: Author.

Amsel, A. (1989). *Behaviorism, neobehaviorism, and cognitivism in learning theory: Historical and contemporary perspectives.* Hillsdale, NJ: Erlbaum.

Andrews, J. D. W., Norcross, J. C., & Halgin, R. P. (1992). Training in psychotherapy integration. In J. C. Norcross & M. R. Goldfried (Eds.), *Handbook of psychotherapy integration* (pp. 563–592). New York: Basic Books.

Argyle, N. (1988). The nature of cognitions in panic disorder. *Behaviour Research and Therapy, 26*(3), 261–264.

Arkowitz, H. (1991). Introductory statement: Psychotherapy integration comes of age. *Journal of Psychotherapy Integration, 1*(1), 1–3.

Arkowitz, H. (1992). Integrative theories of therapy. In D. K. Freedheim (Ed.), *History of psychotherapy: A century of change* (pp. 261–303). Washington, DC: American Psychological Association.

Arkowitz, H., & Hannah, M. T. (1989). Cognitive, behavioral, and psychodynamic therapies: Converging or diverging pathways to change. In A. Freeman, K. M. Simon, L. E. Beutler, & H. Arkowitz (Eds.), *Comprehensive handbook of cognitive therapy* (pp. 143–167). New York: Plenum Press.

Arkowitz, H., & Messer, S. B. (Eds.). (1984). *Psychoanalytic therapy and behavior therapy: Is integration possible?* New York: Plenum Press.

Arnkoff, D. B. (1981). Flexibility in practicing cognitive therapy. In G. Emery, S. D. Hollon, & R. C. Bedrosian (Eds.), *New directions in cognitive therapy* (pp. 203–223). New York: Guilford Press.

Arnkoff, D. B., & Glass, C. R. (1992). Cognitive therapy and psychotherapy integration. In D. F. Freedheim (Ed.), *History of psychotherapy: A century of change* (pp. 657–694). Washington, DC: American Psychological Association.

Ayllon, T., & Azrin, N. H. (1964). Reinforcement and instructions with mental patients. *Journal of the Experimental Analysis of Behavior, 7*, 327–331.

Ayllon, T., & Haughton, E. (1964). Modification of symptomatic verbal behaviour of mental patients. *Behaviour Research and Therapy, 2*, 87–97.

Baer, D. M., Wolf, M. M., & Risley, T. R. (1987). Some still-current dimensions of applied behavior analysis. *Journal of Applied Behavior Analysis, 20*, 313–327.

Barkow, J., Cosmides, L., & Tooby, J. (1992). *The adapted mind: Evolutionary psychology and the generation of culture.* New York: Oxford University Press.

Barlow, D. H. (1988). *Anxiety and its disorders.* New York: Guilford Press.

Barlow, D. H., Craske, M. G., Cerny, J. A., & Klosko, J. S. (1989). Behavioral treatment of panic disorder. *Behavior Therapy, 20*(2), 261–282.

Baron-Cohen, S. (1995). *Mindblindness: An essay on autism and theory of mind.* Cambridge, MA: MIT Press.

Barrowclough, C., & Tarrier, N. (1987). A behavioural family intervention with a schizophrenic patient: A case study. *Behavioural Psychotherapy, 15,* 252–271.

Barrowclough, C., & Tarrier, N. (1992). Interventions with families. In M. Birchwood & N. Tarrier (Eds.), *Innovations in the psychological management of schizophrenia: Assessment, treatment and services* (pp. 79–101). Chichester, England: Wiley.

Baumbacher, G. D. (1989). Signal anxiety and panic attacks. *Psychotherapy: Theory, Research, and Practice, 26*(1), 75–80.

Beck, A. T. (1952). Successful outpatient psychotherapy of a chronic schizophrenic with a delusion based on borrowed guilt. *Psychiatry, 15,* 305–312.

Beck, A. T. (1961). A systematic investigation of depression. *Comprehensive Psychiatry, 2,* 163–170.

Beck, A. T. (1964). Thinking and depression: 2. Theory and therapy. *Archives of General Psychiatry, 10,* 561–571.

Beck, A. T. (1967). *Depression: Causes and treatment.* Philadelphia: University of Pennsylvania Press.

Beck, A. T. (1970a). Cognitive therapy: Nature and relation to behavior therapy. *Behavior Therapy, 1,* 184–200.

Beck, A. T. (1970b). Role of fantasies in psychotherapy and psychopathology. *Journal of Nervous and Mental Disease, 150*(1), 3–17.

Beck, A. T. (1976). *Cognitive therapy and the emotional disorders.* New York: International Universities Press.

Beck, A. T. (1984a). Cognition and therapy [Letter to the editor]. *Archives of General Psychiatry, 41,* 1112–1114.

Beck, A. T. (1984b). Cognitive therapy, behavior therapy, psychoanalysis, and pharmacotherapy: A cognitive continuum. In J. B. W. Williams & R. L. Spitzer (Eds.), *Psychotherapy research: Where are we and where should we go?* (pp. 114–134). New York: Guilford Press.

Beck, A. T. (1985a). Cognitive therapy. In H. I. Kaplan & B. J. Sadock (Eds.), *Comprehensive textbook of psychiatry* (4th ed., Vol. 2, pp. 1432–1438). Baltimore: Williams & Wilkins.

Beck, A. T. (1985b). Theoretical perspectives on clinical anxiety. In A. H. Tuma & J. Maser (Eds.), *Anxiety and the anxiety disorders* (pp. 183–196). Hillsdale, NJ: Erlbaum.

Beck, A. T. (1987a). Cognitive models of depression. *Journal of Cognitive Psychotherapy: An International Quarterly, 1*(1), 5–37.

Beck, A. T. (1987b). Cognitive therapy. In J. K. Zeig (Ed.), *The evolution of psychotherapy* (pp. 149–163). New York: Brunner/Mazel.

Beck, A. T. (1988a). Cognitive approaches to panic disorder: Theory and therapy. In S. Rachman & J. D. Maser (Eds.), *Panic: Psychological perspectives* (pp. 91–109). Hillsdale, NJ: Erlbaum.

Beck, A. T. (1988b). *Love is never enough.* New York: Harper & Row.

Beck, A. T. (1989). Foreword. In J. Scott, J. M. G. Williams, & A. T. Beck (Eds.), *Cognitive therapy in clinical practice: An illustrative casebook* (pp. vii–xv). London: Routledge & Kegan Paul.

Beck, A. T. (1991a). Cognitive therapy as *the* integrative therapy: Comments on Alford and Norcross. *Journal of Psychotherapy Integration, 1*(3), 191–198.

Beck, A. T. (1991b). Cognitive therapy: A 30-year retrospective. *American Psychologist, 46*(4), 368–375.

Beck, A. T. (1992). *Controversial issues in cognitive therapy: Conversation with A. T. Beck* (Cassette Recording No. 920617–280, World Congress of Cognitive Therapy). Richmond Hill, Ontario: Audio Archives of Canada.

Beck, A. T. (1994). Foreword. In D. G. Kingdon & D. Turkington (Eds.), *Cognitive-behavioral therapy of schizophrenia* (pp. v–vii). New York: Guilford Press.

Beck, A. T. (1996). Beyond belief: A theory of modes, personality, and psychopathology. In P. Salkovskis (Ed.), *Frontiers of cognitive therapy* (pp. 1–25). New York: Guilford Press.

Beck, A. T., & Emery, G. (1979). *Cognitive therapy of anxiety and phobic disorders.* Philadelphia: Center for Cognitive Therapy.

Beck, A. T., Emery, G., & Greenberg, R. L. (1985). *Anxiety disorders and phobias: A cognitive perspective.* New York: Basic Books.

Beck, A. T., Freeman, A., & Associates. (1990). *Cognitive therapy of personality disorders.* New York: Guilford Press.

Beck, A. T., & Greenberg, R. L. (1988). Cognitive therapy of panic disorders. In R. E. Hales & A. J. Frances (Eds.), *American Psychiatric Press review of psychiatry* (Vol. 7, pp. 571–583). Washington, DC: American Psychiatric Press.

Beck, A. T., & Hollon, S. (1993). Controversies in cognitive therapy: A dialogue with Aaron T. Beck and Steve Hollon. *Journal of Cognitive Psychotherapy: An International Quarterly, 7*(2), 79–93.

Beck, A. T., Laude, R., & Bohnert, M. (1974). Ideational components of anxiety neurosis. *Archives of General Psychiatry, 31,* 319–325.

Beck, A. T., Newman, C. F., & Wright, F. D. (1989). The Center for Cognitive Therapy at the University of Pennsylvania: Education and training. *The Behavior Therapist, 12*(10), 253–254.

Beck, A. T., Rush, A. J., Shaw, B. F., & Emery, G. (1979). *Cognitive therapy of depression*. New York: Guilford Press.

Beck, A. T., Sokol, L., Clark, D. A., Berchick, R., & Wright, F. (1992). A crossover study of focused cognitive therapy of panic disorder. *American Journal of Psychiatry, 149*, 778–783.

Bentall, R. P., Kinderman, P., & Kaney, S. (1994). The self, attributional processes and abnormal beliefs: Towards a model of persecutory delusions. *Behaviour Research and Therapy, 32*(3), 331–341.

Bergin, A. E., & Garfield, S. L. (1994). Overview, trends, and future issues. In A. E. Bergin & S. L. Garfield (Eds.), *Handbook of psychotherapy and behavior change* (4th ed., pp. 821–830). New York: Wiley.

Beutler, L. E. (1983). *Eclectic psychotherapy: A systematic approach.* Elmsford, NY: Pergamon Press.

Beutler, L. E. (1986). Systematic eclectic psychotherapy. In J. C. Norcross (Ed.), *Handbook of eclectic psychotherapy* (pp. 94–131). New York: Brunner/Mazel.

Biglan, A., Glasgow, R. E., & Singer, G. (1990). The need for a science of larger social units: A contextual approach. *Behavior Therapy, 21*, 195–215.

Bolles, R. C. (1972). Reinforcement, expectancy, and learning. *Psychological Review, 79*(5), 394–409.

Bouton, M. E. (1994). Context, ambiguity, and classical conditioning. *Current Directions in Psychological Science, 3*(2), 49–53.

Brehm, J. W. (1966). *A theory of psychological reactance.* New York: Academic Press.

Brehm, S. S. (1976). *The application of social psychology to clinical practice.* New York: Wiley.

Brewer, W. F. (1974). There is no convincing evidence for operant or classical conditioning in adult humans. In W. Weimer & D. Palermo (Eds.), *Cognition and the symbolic processes* (pp. 1–42). Hillsdale, NJ: Erlbaum.

Calef, R. S., Haupt, A. L., & Choban, M. C. (1994). Delay of reinforcement effects without goal-box confinement. *Psychological Reports, 75*(1), 451–455.

Castonguay, L. G., & Goldfried, M. R. (1994). Psychotherapy integration: An idea whose time has come. *Applied and Preventive Psychology, 3*, 159–172.

Chadwick, P., & Birchwood, M. (1996). *Cognitive therapy with delusions and hallucinations.* New York: Wiley.

Chadwick, P. D. J., & Lowe, C. F. (1990). Measurement and modification of delusional beliefs. *Journal of Consulting and Clinical Psychology, 58*(2), 225–232.

Chance, P. (1988). *Learning and behavior* (2nd ed.). Belmont, CA: Wadsworth.

Clark, D. A. (1995). Perceived limitations of standard cognitive therapy: A consideration of efforts to revise Beck's theory and therapy. *Journal of Cognitive Psychotherapy: An International Quarterly, 9*(3), 153–172.

Clark, D. M. (1986). A cognitive approach to panic. *Behaviour Research and Therapy, 24,* 461–470.

Clark, D. M., Salkovskis, P. M., & Chalkley, A. J. (1985). Respiratory control as a treatment for panic attacks. *Journal of Behavior Therapy and Experimental Psychiatry, 16*(1), 23–30.

Clark, D. M., Salkovskis, P. M., Hackmann, A., Middleton, H., Anastasiades, P., & Gelder, M. (1992). A comparison of cognitive therapy, applied relaxation and imipramine in the treatment of panic disorder. *British Journal of Psychiatry, 164,* 759–769.

Clements, K., & Turpin, G. (1992). Vulnerability models and schizophrenia: The assessment and prediction of relapse. In M. Birchwood & N. Tarrier (Eds.), *Innovations in the psychological management of schizophrenia: Assessment, treatment and services* (pp. 21– 47). Chichester, England: Wiley.

Cloitre, M., Shear, M. K., Cancienne, J., & Zeitlin, S. (1992, November). *Implicit and explicit memory for catastrophic associations to bodily sensation words.* Paper presented at the 26th Annual Meeting of the Association for Advancement of Behavior Therapy, Boston.

Cohen, J., & Stewart, I. (1994). *The collapse of chaos: Discovering simplicity in a complex world.* New York: Viking.

Cohen, J. D., Servan-Schreiber, D., Targ, E., & Spiegel, D. (1992). The fabric of thought disorder: A cognitive neuroscience approach to disturbances in the processing of context in schizophrenia. In D. J. Stein & J. E. Young (Eds.), *Cognitive science and clinical disorders* (pp. 99–127). San Diego: Academic Press.

Coyne, J. C. (1994). Possible contributions of "cognitive science" to the integration of psychotherapy. *Journal of Psychotherapy Integration, 4*(4), 401–416.

Craske, M. G., Brown, T. A., & Barlow, D. H. (1991). Behavioral treatment of panic disorder: A two-year follow-up. *Behavior Therapy, 22,* 289–304.

Craske, M. G., Miller, P. P., Rotunda, R., & Barlow, D. H. (1990). A descriptive report of features of initial unexpected panic attacks in minimal and extensive avoiders. *Behaviour Research and Therapy, 28,* 395–400.

Crick, F. (1994). *The astonishing hypothesis: The scientific search for the soul.* New York: Scribner's.

Crowe, R. R. (1990). Panic disorder: Genetic considerations. *Journal of Psychiatric Research, 24,* 129–134.

Dalgleish, T., & Watts, F. N. (1990). Biases of attention and memory in disorders of anxiety and depression. *Clinical Psychology Review, 10,* 589–604.

Davey, G. (Ed.). (1987a). *Cognitive processes and Pavlovian conditioning in humans.* New York: Wiley.

Davey, G. (1987b). An integration of human and animal models of Pavlovian conditioning: Associations, cognitions, and attributions. In G. Davey (Ed.), *Cognitive processes and Pavlovian conditioning in humans* (pp. 83–114). New York: Wiley.

Davey, G. (1992). Classical conditioning and the acquisition of human fears and phobias: A review and synthesis of the literature. *Advances in Behaviour Research and Therapy, 14,* 29–66.

Dickinson, A. (1980). *Contemporary animal learning theory.* Cambridge, England: Cambridge University Press.

Dickinson, A. (1987). Animal conditioning and learning theory. In H. J. Eysenck & I. Martin (Eds.), *Theoretical foundations of behavior therapy* (pp. 57–79). New York: Plenum Press.

Dingman, C. W., & McGlashan, T. H. (1989). Psychotherapy. In A. S. Bellack (Ed.), *A clinical guide for the treatment of schizophrenia* (pp. 263–282). New York: Plenum Press.

Dobson, K. S. (1989). A meta-analysis of the efficacy of cognitive therapy for depression. *Journal of Consulting and Clinical Psychology, 57*(3), 414–419.

Dougher, M. J. (1993). On the advantages and implications of a radical behavioral treatment of private events. *The Behavior Therapist, 16,* 204–206.

Eifert, G. H., & Evans, I. M. (Eds.). (1990). *Unifying behavior therapy: Contributions of paradigmatic behaviorism.* New York: Springer.

Eifert, G. H., Forsyth, J. P., & Schauss, S. L. (1993). Unifying the field: Developing an integrative paradigm for behavior therapy. *Journal of Behavior Therapy and Experimental Psychiatry, 24*(2), 107–118.

Ellis, A. (1965). An answer to some objections to rational–emotive psychotherapy. *Psychotherapy, 2*(3), 108–111.

Ellis, A. (1993). Reflections on rational–emotive therapy. *Journal of Consulting and Clinical Psychology, 61*(2), 199–201.

Emmelkamp, P. M. G. (1994). Behavior therapy with adults. In A. E. Bergin & S. L. Garfield (Eds.), *Handbook of psychotherapy and behavior change* (4th ed., pp. 379–427). New York: Wiley.

Epstein, S. (1994). Integration of the cognitive and the psychodynamic unconscious. *American Psychologist, 49*(8), 709–724.

Epstein, S., Lipson, A., Holstein, C., & Huh, E. (1992). Irrational reactions to negative outcomes: Evidence for two conceptual systems. *Journal of Personality and Social Psychology, 62*(2), 328–339.

Eysenck, H. J. (1994). The outcome problem in psychotherapy: What have we learned? *Behaviour Research and Therapy, 32*(5), 477–495.

Fishman, D. B., & Franks, C. M. (1992). Evolution and differentiation within behavior therapy: A theoretical and epistemological review. In D. K. Freedheim (Ed.), *History of psychotherapy: A century of change* (pp. 159–196). Washington, DC: American Psychological Association.

Flanagan, O. (1992). *Consciousness reconsidered.* Cambridge, MA: MIT Press.

Flavell, J. H. (1984). Cognitive development during the postinfancy years. In H. W. Stevenson & J. Qicheng (Eds.), *Issues in cognition: Proceedings of a joint conference in psychology* (pp. 1–17). Washington, DC: National Academy of Sciences/American Psychological Association.

Foa, E. B., Ilai, D., McCarthy, P. R., Shoyer, B., & Murdock, T. (1993). Information processing in obsessive–compulsive disorder. *Cognitive Therapy and Research, 17*, 173–189.

Frank, J. D. (1973). *Persuasion and healing* (2nd ed.). Baltimore: Johns Hopkins University Press.

Frank, J. D. (1980). Aristotle as psychotherapist. In M. J. Mahoney (Ed.), *Psychotherapy process: Current issues and future directions* (pp. 335–337). New York: Plenum Press.

Frank, J. D. (1982). Therapeutic components shared by all psychotherapies. In J. Harvey & M. Parks (Eds.), *Psychotherapy research and behavior change: 1981 Master Lecture Series.* Washington, DC: American Psychological Association.

Franks, C. M. (1984). A rejoinder to Leon Salzman. In H. Arkowitz & S. B. Messer (Eds.), *Psychoanalytic therapy and behavior therapy: Is integration possible?* (pp. 253–254). New York: Plenum Press.

Freeman, W. J. (1991). The physiology of perception. *Scientific American, 264*, 78–85.

Freud, S. (1950). Mourning and melancholia. In E. Jones (Ed.), *Sigmund Freud: Collected papers* (Vol. 4, pp. 152–172). London: Hogarth Press. (Original work published 1917)

Fritze, J., Forthner, B., Schmitt, B., & Thaler, U. (1988). Cognitive training adjunctive to pharmacotherapy in schizophrenia and depression: A pilot study on the lateralization hypothesis of schizophrenia and depression, and cognitive therapy as adjunctive treatment. *Neuropsychobiology, 19,* 45–50.

Garfield, E. (1992, November). A citationist perspective of psychology: Most cited papers, 1986–1990. *APS Observer,* pp. 8–9.

Garfield, S. L. (1980). *Psychotherapy: An eclectic approach.* New York: Wiley.

Garfield, S. L. (1986). An eclectic psychotherapy. In J. C. Norcross (Ed.), *Handbook of eclectic psychotherapy* (pp. 132–162). New York: Brunner/Mazel.

Gelder, M. G. (1986). Panic attacks: New approaches to an old problem. *British Journal of Psychiatry, 149,* 346–352.

Gelder, M. G., & Marks, I. M. (1966). Severe agoraphobia: A controlled prospective trial of behaviour therapy. *British Journal of Psychiatry, 112,* 309–319.

Gilbert, P. (1989). *Human nature and suffering.* Hillsdale, NJ: Erlbaum.

Gluhoski, V. L. (1994). Misconceptions of cognitive therapy. *Psychotherapy, 31*(4), 594–600.

Goldfried, M. R. (1980). Toward the delineation of therapeutic change principles. *American Psychologist, 35,* 991–999.

Goldfried, M. R., & Davison, G. C. (1976). *Clinical behavior therapy.* New York: Holt, Rinehart & Winston.

Goldfried, M. R., & Newman, C. (1986). Psychotherapy integration: An historical perspective. In J. C. Norcross (Ed.), *Handbook of eclectic psychotherapy* (pp. 25–61). New York: Brunner/Mazel.

Goldman, A. I. (1993). Consciousness, folk psychology, and cognitive science. *Consciousness and Cognition, 2,* 364–382.

Green, M. F. (1993). Cognitive remediation in schizophrenia: Is it time yet? *American Journal of Psychiatry, 150,* 178–187.

Greenberg, L. S., Elliott, R. K., & Lietaer, G. (1994). Research on experiential psychotherapies. In A. E. Bergin & S. L. Garfield (Eds.), *Handbook of psychotherapy and behavior change* (4th ed., pp. 509–539). New York: Wiley.

Greenwood, V. B. (1983). Cognitive therapy with the young adult chronic patient. In A. Freeman (Ed.), *Cognitive therapy with couples and groups* (pp. 183–198). New York: Plenum Press.

Grencavage, L. M., & Norcross, J. C. (1990). Where are the commonalities among the therapeutic common factors? *Professional Psychology: Research and Practice, 21*(5), 372–378.

Haaga, D. A. F. (1986). A review of the common principles approach to integration of psychotherapies. *Cognitive Therapy and Research, 10*(5), 527–538.

Haaga, D. A. F., & Beck, A. T. (1995). Perspectives on depressive realism: Implications for cognitive theory of depression. *Behaviour Research and Therapy, 33*(1), 41–48.

Haaga, D. A. F., Dyck, M. J., & Ernst, D. (1991). Empirical status of cognitive theory of depression. *Psychological Bulletin, 110*, 215–236.

Halford, W. K. (1991). Beyond expressed emotion: Behavioral assessment of family interaction associated with the course of schizophrenia. *Behavioral Assessment, 13*, 199–123.

Hand, I., Lamontagne, Y., & Marks, I. M. (1974). Group exposure (flooding) *in vivo* for agoraphobics. *British Journal of Psychiatry, 124*, 588–602.

Harris, M. J. (1994). Self-fulfilling prophecies in the clinical context: Review and implications for clinical practice. *Applied and Preventive Psychology, 3*, 145–158.

Harrow, M., & Miller, J. G. (1980). Schizophrenic thought disorders and impaired perspective. *Journal of Abnormal Psychology, 89*, 717–727.

Hatfield, A. B. (1989). Patients' accounts of stress and coping in schizophrenia. *Hospital and Community Psychiatry, 40*, 1141–1145.

Hayes, L. J., & Chase, P. N. (1991). *Dialogues on verbal behavior.* Reno, NV: Context Press.

Hayes, S. C., & Wilson, K. G. (1993). Some applied implications of a contemporary behavior-analytic account of verbal events. *The Behavior Analyst, 16*, 283–301.

Heinssen, R. K., & Victor, B. J. (1994). Cognitive-behavioral treatments for schizophrenia: Evolving rehabilitation techniques. In W. Spaulding (Ed.), *Cognitive technology in psychiatric rehabilitation* (pp. 1–44). Lincoln: University of Nebraska Press.

Henry, W. P., Strupp, H. H., Schacht, T. E., & Gaston, L. (1994). Psychodynamic approaches. In A. E. Bergin & S. L. Garfield (Eds.), *Handbook of psychotherapy and behavior change* (4th ed., pp. 467–508). New York: Wiley.

Hibbert, G. A. (1984). Ideational components of anxiety: Their origin and content. *British Journal of Psychiatry, 144,* 618–624.

Himadi, B., Osteen, F., & Crawford, E. (1993). Delusional verbalizations and beliefs. *Behavioral Residential Treatment, 8,* 229–242.

Himadi, B., Osteen, F., Kaiser, A. J., & Daniel, K. (1991). Assessment of delusional beliefs during the modification of delusional verbalizations. *Behavioral Residential Treatment, 6*(5), 355–366.

Holden, C. (1994). Scholars defend bell curve. *Science, 266,* 1811.

Hole, R. W., Rush, A. J., & Beck, A. T. (1979). A cognitive investigation of schizophrenic delusions. *Psychiatry, 42,* 312–319.

Holland, P. C., & Rescorla, R. A. (1975). The effect of two ways of devaluing the unconditioned stimulus after first- and second-order appetitive conditioning. *Journal of Experimental Psychology: Animal Behavior Processes, 1,* 355–363.

Holland, P. C., & Straub, J. J. (1979). Differential effects of two ways of devaluing the unconditioned stimulus after Pavlovian appetitive conditioning. *Journal of Experimental Psychology: Animal Behavior Processes, 5,* 65–78.

Hollon, S. D., & Beck, A. T. (1994). Cognitive and cognitive-behavioral therapies. In A. E. Bergin & S. L. Garfield (Eds.), *Handbook of psychotherapy and behavior change* (4th ed., pp. 428–466). New York: Wiley.

Hollon, S. D., DeRubeis, R. J., & Seligman, M. E. P. (1992). Cognitive therapy and the prevention of depression. *Applied and Preventive Psychology, 1,* 89–95.

Hollon, S. D., & Garber, J. (1990). Cognitive therapy for depression: A social cognitive perspective. *Personality and Social Psychology Bulletin, 16,* 58–73.

Hollon, S. D., & Najavits, L. (1988). Review of empirical studies of cognitive therapy. In A. J. Frances & R. E. Hales (Eds.), *American Psychiatric Press review of psychiatry* (Vol. 7, pp. 643–666). Washington, DC: American Psychiatric Press.

Horowitz, M. J. (1991). States, schemas, and control: General theories for psychotherapy integration. *Journal of Psychotherapy Integration, 1*(2), 85–102.

Jacobson, N. S. (1985a). The role of observational measures in behavior therapy outcome research. *Behavioral Assessment, 7,* 297–308.

Jacobson, N. S. (1985b). Uses versus abuses of observational measures. *Behavioral Assessment, 7,* 323–330.

Jacobson, N. S. (1992). Behavioral couple therapy: A new beginning. *Behavior Therapy, 23*(4), 493–506.

Johnson, S. M., & White, G. (1971). Self-observation as an agent of behavioral change. *Behavior Therapy, 2*, 488–497.

Kazdin, A. E. (1978). *History of behavior modification: Experimental foundation of contemporary research.* Baltimore: University Park Press.

Kazdin, A. E. (1984). Integration of psychodynamic and behavioral psychotherapies: Conceptual versus empirical synthesis. In H. Arkowitz & S. B. Messer (Eds.), *Psychoanalytic therapy and behavior therapy: Is integration possible?* (pp. 139–170). New York: Plenum Press.

Kelly, G. A. (1955). *The psychology of personal constructs* (2 vols.). New York: Norton.

Kenardy, J., Evans, L., & Oei, T. P. S. (1988). The importance of cognitions in panic attacks. *Behavior Therapy, 19*(3), 471–483.

Kendall, P. C. (1977). On the efficacious use of verbal self-instructional procedures with children. *Cognitive Therapy and Research, 1*, 331–341.

Kendall, P. C. (1993). Cognitive-behavioral therapies with youth: Guiding theory, current status, and emerging developments. *Journal of Consulting and Clinical Psychology, 61*(2), 235–247.

Kendall, P. C., & Braswell, L. (1985). *Cognitive-behavioral therapy for impulsive children.* New York: Guilford Press.

Kendall, P. C., & Finch, A. J., Jr. (1976). A cognitive-behavioral treatment for impulse control: A case study. *Journal of Consulting and Clinical Psychology, 44*, 852–857.

Kihlstrom, J. F. (1987). The cognitive unconscious. *Science, 237*, 1445–1452.

Kimble, G. A. (1961). *Hilgard and Marquis' conditioning and learning.* New York: Appleton-Century-Crofts.

Kingdon, D. G., & Turkington, D. (1991a). A role for cognitive-behavioural strategies in schizophrenia? *Social Psychiatry and Psychiatric Epidemiology, 26*, 101–103.

Kingdon, D. G., & Turkington, D. (1991b). The use of cognitive behavior therapy with a normalizing rationale in schizophrenia. *Journal of Nervous and Mental Disease, 179*(4), 207–211.

Klein, D. F. (1981). Anxiety reconceptualized. In D. F. Klein & J. G. Rabkin (Eds.), *Anxiety: New research and changing concepts* (pp. 235–263). New York: Raven Press.

Knell, S. M. (1990, November). *Cognitive-behavioral play therapy.* Paper presented at the annual meeting of the Association for Advancement of Behavior Therapy, San Francisco.

Kreitler, H., & Kreitler, S. (1982). The theory of cognitive orientation: Widening the scope of behavior prediction. In B. Maher & W. B. Maher (Eds.), *Progress in experimental personality research* (pp. 101–169). New York: Academic Press.

Kreitler, H., & Kreitler, S. (1990). Cognitive primacy, cognitive behavior guidance, and their implications for cognitive therapy. *Journal of Cognitive Psychotherapy: An International Quarterly, 4*(2), 151–169.

Laing, R. D. (1967). *The politics of experience.* New York: Pantheon Books.

Lazarus, A. A. (1967). In support of technical eclecticism. *Psychological Reports, 21,* 415–416.

Lazarus, A. A. (1989). *The practice of multimodal therapy.* Baltimore: Johns Hopkins University Press.

Lazarus, A. A. (1995a). Different types of eclecticism and integration: Let's be aware of the dangers. *Journal of Psychotherapy Integration, 5*(1), 27–39.

Lazarus, A. A. (1995b). Integration and clinical verisimilitude [Review of *Comprehensive handbook of psychotherapy integration*]. *Clinical Psychology: Science and Practice, 2*(4), 399–402.

Lazarus, A. A., & Messer, S. B. (1991). Does chaos prevail? An exchange on technical eclecticism and assimilative integration. *Journal of Psychotherapy Integration, 1*(2), 143–158.

Lazarus, R. S. (1991a). Cognition and motivation in emotion. *American Psychologist, 46*(4), 352–367.

Lazarus, R. S. (1991b). *Emotion and adaptation.* New York: Oxford University Press.

Lazarus, R. S. (1991c). Progress on a cognitive–motivational–relational theory of emotion. *American Psychologist, 46*(8), 819–834.

Lazarus, R. S., & Folkman, S. (1986). Cognitive theories of stress and the issue of circularity. In M. H. Appley & R. Trumbull (Eds.), *Dynamics of stress: Physiological, psychological, and social perspectives* (pp. 63–80). New York: Plenum Press.

Leahy, R. L. (1995). Cognitive development and cognitive therapy. *Journal of Cognitive Psychotherapy: An International Quarterly, 9*(3), 173–184.

Leakey, R. (1994). *The origin of humankind.* New York: Basic Books.

Liberman, R. P., Teigen, J., Patterson, R., & Baker, V. (1973). Reducing delusional speech in chronic paranoid schizophrenics. *Journal of Applied Behavior Analysis, 6,* 57–64.

Liebert, R. M., & Spiegler, M. D. (1987). *Personality: Strategies and issues* (5th ed.). Homewood, IL: Dorsey Press.

Loeb, A., Beck, A. T., & Diggory, J. (1971). Differential effects of success and failure on depressed and nondepressed patients. *Journal of Nervous and Mental Disease, 152,* 106–114.

Logan, A., Larkin, K., & Whittal, M. (1992, November). *Threat cues in non-clinical anxiety: Specificity of attention and interpretation.* Paper presented at the 26th annual meeting of the Association for Advancement of Behavior Therapy, Boston.

Lyon, H. M., Kaney, S., & Bentall, R. P. (1994). The defensive function of persecutory delusions: Evidence from attribution tasks. *British Journal of Psychiatry, 164,* 637–646.

Mackintosh, N. J. (1983). *Conditioning and associative learning.* Oxford: Oxford University Press.

MacLeod, C. (1991). Clinical anxiety and the selective encoding of threatening information. *International Review of Psychiatry, 3,* 279–292.

MacLeod, C., & Mathews, A. M. (1991). Cognitive-experimental approaches to the emotional disorders. In P. R. Martin (Ed.), *Handbook of behavior therapy and psychological science: An integrative approach* (pp. 116–150). Elmsford, NY: Pergamon Press.

Mahoney, M. J. (1989). Holy epistemology! Construing the constructions of the constructivists. *Canadian Psychology, 30*(2), 187–188.

Mahoney, M. J. (1993). Introduction to special section: Theoretical developments in the cognitive psychotherapies. *Journal of Consulting and Clinical Psychology, 61*(2), 187–193.

Mahoney, M. J., & Mahoney, K. (1976). *Permanent weight control.* New York: Norton.

Malott, R. W. (1980). *Rule-governed behavior and the achievement of evasive goals: A theoretical analysis.* Unpublished manuscript, Western Michigan University, Department of Psychology, Kalamazoo.

Manicas, P. T., & Secord, P. F. (1983). Implications for psychology of the new philosophy of science. *American Psychologist, 38*(4), 399–413.

Margraf, J., Ehlers, A., & Roth, W. T. (1987). Panic attack associated with perceived heart rate acceleration: A case report. *Behavior Therapy, 18,* 84–89.

Marks, I. M. (1971). Phobic disorders four years after treatment. *British Journal of Psychiatry, 118,* 683–688.

Marks, I. M. (1987a). Behavioral aspects of panic disorder. *American Journal of Psychiatry, 144,* 1160–1165.

Marks, I. M. (1987b). *Fears, phobias, and rituals: Panic, anxiety, and their disorders.* New York: Oxford University Press.

Marks, I. M., & Gelder, M. G. (1966). Different ages of onset in varieties of phobia. *American Journal of Psychiatry, 123*(2), 218– 221.

Marks, I. M., Gray, S., Cohen, D., Hill, R., Mawson, D., Ramm, E., & Stern, R. S. (1983). Imipramine and brief therapist-aided exposure in agoraphobics having self-exposure homework. *Archives of General Psychiatry, 40,* 153–162.

Martin, I., & Levey, A. B. (1985). Conditioning, evaluations and cognitions: An axis of integration. *Behaviour Research and Therapy, 23*(2), 167–175.

Marzillier, J. S., & Birchwood, M. J. (1981). Behavioral treatment of cognitive disorders. In L. Michelson, M. Hersen, & S. Turner (Eds.), *Future perspectives in behavior therapy* (pp. 131–159). New York: Plenum Press.

McGlashan, T. H., Heinssen, R. K., & Fenton, W. S. (1989). Psychosocial treatment of negative symptoms in schizophrenia. In N. C. Andreasen (Ed.), *Modern problems in pharmacopsychiatry: Vol. 24. Schizophrenia: Positive and negative symptoms and syndromes* (pp. 175–200). Basel: Karger.

McNally, R. J. (1990). Psychological approaches to panic disorder: A review. *Psychological Bulletin, 108*(3), 403–419.

McNally, R. J. (1995). Automaticity and the anxiety disorders. *Behaviour Research and Therapy, 33*(7), 747–754.

Meichenbaum, D. H. (1976). Toward a cognitive theory of self-control. In G. E. Schwartz & D. Shapiro (Eds.), *Consciousness and self-regulation* (pp. 223–260). New York: Plenum Press.

Meichenbaum, D. H. (1993). Changing conceptions of cognitive behavior modification: Retrospect and prospect. *Journal of Consulting and Clinical Psychology, 61*(2), 202–204.

Meichenbaum, D. H., & Cameron, R. (1973). Training schizophrenics to talk to themselves: A means of developing attentional controls. *Behavior Therapy, 4,* 515–534.

Meichenbaum, D. H., & Gilmore, J. B. (1984). The nature of unconscious processes: A cognitive-behavioral perspective. In K. S. Bowers & D. Meichenbaum (Eds.), *The unconscious reconsidered* (pp. 273–298). New York: Wiley.

Messer, S. B. (1987). Can the tower of Babel be completed? A critique of the common language proposal. *Journal of Integrative and Eclectic Psychotherapy, 6,* 195–199.

Michelson, L. K., & Marchione, K. (1991). Behavioral, cognitive, and pharmacological treatments of panic disorder with agoraphobia: Critique and synthesis. *Journal of Consulting and Clinical Psychology, 59*(1), 100–114.

Milton, F., Patwa, V. K., & Hafner, R. J. (1978). Confrontation versus belief modification in persistently deluded patients. *British Journal of Medical Psychology, 51,* 127–130.

Mineka, S., & Sutton, S. K. (1992). Cognitive biases and the emotional disorders. *Psychological Science, 3*(1), 65–69.

Mischel, W. (1961). Preferences for delayed reinforcement and social responsibility. *Journal of Abnormal and Social Psychology, 62,* 1–7.

Mischel, W. (1974). Processes in delay of gratification. In L. Berkowitz (Ed.), *Advances in experimental social psychology* (Vol. 7, pp. 249–292). New York: Academic Press.

Mischel, W., & Patterson, C. J. (1976). Substantive and structural elements of effective plans for self-control. *Journal of Personality and Social Psychology, 34,* 942–950.

Monahan, J., & O'Leary, K. D. (1971). Effects of self-instruction on rule-breaking behavior. *Psychological Reports, 29,* 1059–1066.

Moore, J. (1984). On privacy, causes, and contingencies. *The Behavior Analyst, 7,* 3–16.

Moretti, M. M., & Shaw, B. F. (1989). Automatic and dysfunctional cognitive processes in depression. In J. S. Uleman & J. A. Bargh (Eds.), *Unintended thought* (pp. 383–421). New York: Guilford Press.

Morrison, A. P. (1994). Cognitive behaviour therapy for auditory hallucinations without concurrent medication: A single case. *Behavioural and Cognitive Psychotherapy, 22,* 259–264.

Morrison, A. P., Haddock, G., & Tarrier, N. (in press). Intrusive thoughts and auditory hallucinations: A cognitive approach. *Behavioural and Cognitive Psychotherapy.*

Mowrer, O. H., & Ullman, A. D. (1945). Time as a determinant in integrative learning. *Psychological Review, 52,* 61–90.

Neimeyer, R. A. (1993). An appraisal of constructivist psychotherapies. *Journal of Consulting and Clinical Psychology, 61*(2), 221–234.

Norcross, J. C. (1986). Eclectic psychotherapy: An introduction and overview. In J. C. Norccross (Ed.), *Handbook of eclectic psychotherapy* (pp. 3–24). New York: Brunner/Mazel.

Norcross, J. C. (1988). The exclusivity myth and the equifinality principle in psychotherapy. *Journal of Integrative and Eclectic Psychotherapy, 7*(4), 415–421.

Norcross, J. C. (1990). Commentary: Eclecticism misrepresented and integration misunderstood. *Psychotherapy, 27,* 297–300.

Norcross, J. C., Alford, B. A., & DeMichele, J. T. (1992). The future of psychotherapy: Delphi data and concluding observations. *Psychotherapy, 29*(1), 150–158.

Norcross, J. C., & Prochaska, J. O. (1988). A study of eclectic (and integrative) views revisited. *Professional Psychology: Research and Practice, 19,* 170–174.

Norcross, J. C., & Thomas, B. L. (1988). What's stopping us now?: Obstacles to psychotherapy integration. *Journal of Integrative and Eclectic Psychotherapy, 7,* 74–80.

Novaco, R. (1975). *Anger control: The development and evaluation of an experimental treatment.* Lexington, MA: D. C. Heath.

O'Donohue, W., & Krasner, L. (Eds.). (1995). *Theories of behavior therapy: Exploring behavior change.* Washington, DC: American Psychological Association.

O'Leary, K. D. (1968). The effects of self-instructions on immoral behavior. *Journal of Experimental Child Psychology, 6,* 297–301.

Oltmanns, T. F., & Mineka, S. (1992). Morton Prince on anxiety disorders: Intellectual antecedents of the cognitive approach to panic? *Journal of Abnormal Psychology, 101*(4), 607–610.

Omer, H., & London, P. (1988). Metamorphosis in psychotherapy: End of the systems era. *Psychotherapy, 25,* 171–180.

Oppenheimer, J. R. (1956). Analogy in science. *American Psychologist, 11,* 127–135.

Pavlov, I. P. (1927). *Conditioned reflexes.* Oxford: Oxford University Press.

Pepper, S. C. (1963). A proposal for a world hypothesis. *The Monist, 47*(2), 267–286.

Perris, C. (1989). *Cognitive therapy with schizophrenic patients.* New York: Guilford Press.

Persons, J. B. (1989). *Cognitive therapy in practice: A case formulation approach.* New York: Norton.

Popper, K. R. (1959). *The logic of scientific discovery.* New York: Basic Books.

Powers, W. T. (1992). A cognitive control system. In R. L. Levine & H. E. Fitzgerald (Eds.), *Analysis of dynamic psychological systems: Methods and applications* (Vol. 2, pp. 327–340). New York: Plenum Press.

Pretzer, J. L., & Beck, A. T. (1996). A cognitive theory of personality disorders. In J. F. Clarkin (Ed.), *Major theories of personality disorder* (pp. 36–105). New York: Guilford Press.

Prochaska, J. O., & DiClemente, C. C. (1982). Transtheoretical therapy: Toward a more integrated model of change. *Psychotherapy: Theory, Research, and Practice, 19,* 276–288.

Prochaska, J. O., & DiClemente, C. C. (1984). *The transtheoretical approach: Crossing the traditional boundaries of therapy.* Homewood, IL: Dow Jones-Irvin.

Prochaska, J. O., & Norcross, J. C. (1994). *Systems of psychotherapy: A transtheoretical approach.* Pacific Grove, CA: Brooks/Cole.

Rachlin, H. (1992). Teleological behaviorism. *American Psychologist, 47*(11), 1371–1382.

Rachman, S. J. (1990). *Fear and courage.* New York: W. H. Freeman.

Rapee, R. M. (1987). The psychological treatment of panic attacks: Theoretical conceptualization and review of evidence. *Clinical Psychology Review, 7,* 427–438.

Rapee, R. M. (1991a). The conceptual overlap between cognition and conditioning in clinical psychology. *Clinical Psychology Review, 11,* 193–203.

Rapee, R. M. (1991b). Panic disorder. *International Review of Psychiatry, 3,* 141–149.

Rapee, R. M., Telfer, L. A., & Barlow, D. H. (1991). The role of safety cues in mediating the response to inhalants of CO-sub-2 in agoraphobics. *Behaviour Research and Therapy, 29,* 353–355.

Reiss, S. (1980). Pavlovian conditioning and human fear: An expectancy model. *Behavior Therapy, 11,* 380–396.

Renner, K. E. (1964). Delay of reinforcement: A historical perspective. *Psychological Bulletin, 61,* 341–361.

Rescorla, R. A. (1987). A Pavlovian analysis of goal-directed behavior. *American Psychologist, 42,* 119–129.

Rescorla, R. A. (1988). Pavlovian conditioning: It's not what you think it is. *American Psychologist, 43*(3), 151–160.

Rescorla, R. A., & Holland, P. C. (1977). Behavioral studies of associative learning in animals. *Annual Review of Psychology, 33,* 265–308.

Revusky, S. H. (1977). Learning as a general process with an emphasis on data from feeding experiments. In N. W. Milgram, L. Krames, & T. M. Alloway (Eds.), *Food aversion learning* (pp. 1–51). New York: Plenum Press.

Riskind, J. H. (1991). A set of cognitive priming interventions for cognitive therapy homework exercises. *The Behavior Therapist, 14,* 43–44.

Robins, C. J., & Hayes, A. M. (1993). An appraisal of cognitive therapy. *Journal of Consulting and Clinical Psychology, 61*(2), 205–214.

Ross, A. O. (1987). *Personality: The scientific study of complex human behavior.* New York: Holt, Rinehart & Winston.

Rust, J. (1990). Delusions, irrationality and cognitive science. *Philosophical Psychology, 3*(1), 123–138.

Ryle, A. (1982). *Psychotherapy: A cognitive integration of theory and practice.* London: Academic Press.

Safran, J. (1984). Assessing the cognitive–interpersonal cycle. *Cognitive Therapy and Research, 8,* 333–347.

Safran, J. D. (1984). Some implications of Sullivan's interpersonal theory for cognitive therapy. In M. A. Reda & M. J. Mahoney (Eds.), *Cognitive psychotherapies: Recent developments in theory, research and practice* (pp. 251–272). Cambridge, MA: Ballinger.

Safran, J. D., & Greenberg, L. S. (1986). Hot cognition and psychotherapy process: An information-processing ecological approach. In P. C. Kendall (Ed.), *Advances in cognitive-behavioral research and therapy* (Vol. 5, pp. 143–177). New York: Plenum Press.

Salkovskis, P. M., & Clark, D. M. (1986). Respiratory control in the treatment of panic attacks: Replication and extension with current measurement of behaviour and pCO-sub-2. *British Journal of Psychiatry, 148,* 526–532.

Salkovskis, P. M., & Clark, D. M. (1990). Affective responses to hyperventilation: A test of the cognitive model of panic. *Behaviour Research and Therapy, 28,* 51–61.

Salkovskis, P. M., & Clark, D. M. (1991). Treatment of panic attacks using cognitive therapy without exposure or breathing retraining. *Behaviour Research and Therapy, 29,* 161–166.

Salzman, I. J. (1951). Delay of reward and human verbal learning. *Journal of Experimental Psychology, 41,* 437–439.

Sargent, M. (1990, June). NIMH report: Panic disorder. *Hospital and Community Psychiatry, 41,* 621–623.

Schacht, T. E. (1984). The varieties of integrative experience. In H. Arkowitz & S. B. Messer (Eds.), *Psychoanalytic therapy and behavior therapy: Is integration possible?* (pp. 107–131). New York: Plenum Press.

Scott, J. (1989). Cancer patients. In J. Scott, J. M. G. Williams, & A. T. Beck (Eds.), *Cognitive therapy in clinical practice: An illustrative casebook* (pp. 103–126). London: Routledge & Kegan Paul.

Searle, J. R. (1990). Is the brain a digital computer? *American Philosophical Association Proceedings, 64*(3), 21–37.

Searle, J. R. (1992). *The rediscovery of the mind.* Cambridge: MIT Press.

Searle, J. R. (1993). The problem of consciousness. *Consciousness and Cognition, 2,* 310–319.

Searle, J. R. (1994). The problem of consciousness. In A. Revonsuo

& M. Kamppinen (Eds.), *Consciousness in philosophy and cognitive neuroscience* (pp. 93–104). Hillsdale, NJ: Erlbaum.

Segal, Z. V. (1988). Appraisal of the self-schema construct in cognitive models of depression. *Psychological Bulletin, 103,* 147–162.

Seligman, M. E. P. (1971). Phobias and preparedness. *Behavior Therapy, 2,* 307–320.

Seligman, M. E. P. (1988). Competing theories of panic. In J. S. Rachman & J. D. Maser (Eds.), *Panic: Psychological perspectives* (pp. 321–329). Hillsdale, NJ: Erlbaum.

Shybut, J. (1968). Delay of gratification and severity of psychological disturbance among hospitalized psychiatric inpatients. *Journal of Consulting and Clinical Psychology, 32,* 462–468.

Siddle, D. A. T., & Remington, B. (1987). Latent inhibition and human Pavlovian conditioning: Research and relevance. In G. Davey (Ed.), *Cognitive processes and Pavlovian conditioning in humans* (pp. 115–146). New York: Wiley.

Skinner, B. F. (1963). Behaviorism at fifty. *Science, 140,* 951–958.

Skinner, B. F. (1969). *Contingencies of reinforcement: A theoretical analysis.* New York: Appleton-Century-Crofts.

Skinner, B. F. (1981). Selection by consequences. *Science, 213,* 501–504.

Smith, R. J. (1964). A note on rational–emotive psychotherapy: Some problems. *Psychotherapy, 1*(4), 151–153.

Sokol, L., Beck, A. T., Greenberg, R. L., Berchick, R. J., & Wright, F. D. (1989). Cognitive therapy of panic disorder: A non-pharmacological alternative. *Journal of Nervous and Mental Disease, 177,* 711–716.

Spaulding, W. D., Garbin, C. P., & Crinean, W. J. (1989). The logical and psychometric prerequisites for cognitive therapy of schizophrenia. *British Journal of Psychiatry, 155,* 69–73.

Spaulding, W. D., Storms, L., Goodrich, V., & Sullivan, M. (1986). Applications of experimental psychopathology in psychiatric rehabilitation. *Schizophrenia Bulletin, 12,* 560–577.

Staats, A. W. (1991). Unified positivism and unification psychology: Fad or new field? *American Psychologist, 46*(9), 899–912.

Stahl, J. R., & Leitenberg, H. (1976). Behavioral treatment of the chronic mental hospital patient. In H. Leitenberg (Ed.), *Handbook of behavior modification and behavior therapy* (pp. 211–241). Englewood Cliffs, NJ: Prentice-Hall.

Stein, D. J., & Young, J. E. (Eds.). (1992). *Cognitive science and clinical disorders.* San Diego: Academic Press.

Sternberg, R. J. (1993). Parts is parts, but isn't there more to the whole? *Contemporary Psychology, 38*(12), 1271–1274.

Sternberg, R. J. (1994). PRSVL: An integrative framework for understanding mind in context. In R. J. Sternberg (Ed.), *Mind in context: Interactionist perspectives on human intelligence* (pp. 218– 232). New York: Cambridge University Press.

Strupp, H. H., & Binder, J. (1984). *Psychotherapy in a new key.* New York: Basic Books.

Tarrier, N. (1992). Management and modification of residual positive psychotic symptoms. In M. Birchwood & N. Tarrier (Eds.), *Innovations in the psychological management of schizophrenia: Assessment, treatment and services* (pp. 147–169). Chichester, England: Wiley.

Tarrier, N., Beckett, R., Harwood, S., Baker, A., Yusupoff, L., & Ugarteburu, I. (1993). A trial of two cognitive behavioural methods of treating drug-resistant residual psychotic symptoms in schizophrenic patients: I. Outcome. *British Journal of Psychiatry, 162,* 524–532.

Teasdale, J. D., & Barnard, P. J. (1993). *Affect, cognition, and change: Re-modeling depressive thought.* Hillsdale, NJ: Erlbaum.

Testa, T. J. (1974). Causal relationships and the acquisition of avoidance response. *Psychological Review, 81,* 491–505.

Wachtel, P. L. (1977). *Psychoanalysis and behavior therapy: Toward an integration.* New York: Basic Books.

Wachtel, P. L. (1987). *Action and insight.* New York: Guilford Press.

Wasylenki, D. A. (1992). Psychotherapy of schizophrenia revisited. *Hospital and Community Psychiatry, 43,* 123–127.

Watson, J. B., & Rayner, R. (1920). Conditioned emotional reactions. *Journal of Experimental Psychology, 3,* 1–14.

Watts, F. N., Powell, G. E., & Austin, S. V. (1973). The modification of abnormal beliefs. *British Journal of Medical Psychology, 46,* 359–363.

Wegner, D. M. (1994). Ironic processes of mental control. *Psychological Review, 101,* 34–52.

Weishaar, M. E. (1993). *Aaron T. Beck.* London: Sage.

Werner, G., Reitboeck, H. J., & Eckhorn, R. (1993). Construction of concepts by the nervous system: From neurons to cognition. *Behavioral Science, 38,* 114–123.

Whaley, D. L. (1978). *Origins of hope and dread.* Unpublished manuscript, North Texas State University.

White, P. A. (1990). Ideas about causation in philosophy and psychology. *Psychological Bulletin, 108*(1), 3–18.

Wincze, J. P., Leitenberg, H., & Agras, W. S. (1972). The effects of token reinforcement and feedback on the delusional verbal behavior of chronic paranoid schizophrenics. *Journal of Applied Behavior Analysis, 5,* 247–262.

Wolfe, B. E. (1994). Introduction to special issue on cognitive science and psychotherapy. *Journal of Psychotherapy Integration, 4*(4), 285–289.

Wolpe, J., & Rowan, V. C. (1988). Panic disorder: A product of classical conditioning. *Behaviour Research and Therapy, 26*(6), 441–450.

Wright, J. H., & Davis, D. (1994). The therapeutic relationship in cognitive-behavioral therapy: Patient perceptions and therapist responses. *Cognitive and behavioral practice, 1,* 25–45.

Yeaton, W. H., & Sechrest, L. (1981). Critical dimensions in the choice and maintenance of successful treatments: Strength, integrity, and effectiveness. *Journal of Consulting and Clinical Psychology, 49,* 156–167.

Young, J. E. (1990). *Cognitive therapy for personality disorders: A schema-focused approach.* Sarasota, FL: Professional Resource Exchange.

Zubin, J., & Spring, B. (1977). Vulnerability: A new view of schizophrenia. *Journal of Abnormal Psychology, 86,* 103–126.

# Index

Abreative techniques, 91
Adaptive processes
  and anxiety, 21, 22
  schemas function in, 29
Agoraphobia (*see* Panic disorder)
Analogies, 33–36, 43, 44
Animal models, 132, 133
Anxiety conditioning, 116, 117
Anxiety disorders, 20–22 (*see also*
  Panic disorder)
  automatic cognitive processing in,
    20
  transfixed attentional resources in,
    20–22
Anxiety neurosis, in DSM-II, 121
Arbitrary inferences, 145–147
Arousal, primacy question, panic,
  133–135
Attentional resources
  in anxiety disorders, 20–22
  in panic disorder, 20–22, 122–125
  theoretical aspects, 20–22
Automatic cognitive system, 65–70
Automatic thoughts, 18–20
  anxiety disorders role, theory, 21,
    123, 124
  cognitive theory axiom, 17
  expressed emotion role, 152–154
  internal and external variables, 107
  in panic disorder, 123–125
  theoretical aspects, 18–22, 107

Behavioral techniques
  cognitive therapy relationship, 60–
    63, 91, 130, 131
  in delusional beliefs, 60–63

in panic disorder, 130, 131
  therapeutic relationship in, 79
  verbal behavior focus of, 61–63
Behavioral theories (*see also* Condi-
    tioning models)
  and causal analysis, 39, 40
  cognitive theory differences, 60–63
  and consciousness, 52, 53
  instructional training interpretation,
    57, 58
  levels of function in, 66, 67
  paradigm shift from, 60–63
  and temporal-consequences
    conflicts, 51–53

Catastrophic misperceptions
  and cognitive theory, 100–102
  in panic disorder, 100, 101, 122–
    125, 129, 130
  Pavlovian and cognitive theory of,
    129, 130
  postconditioning revaluation, 132
  primacy question, panic etiology,
    134, 135
Causes, 39–41
  in behavioral theory, 39, 40
  in cognitive theory, 39–41
  radical behavioral interpretation,
    40, 41
Circular theory, 36, 37
Classical conditioning
  and anxiety, 116–118
  cognitive theory relationship, 64,
    65, 126–128
  constructivist perspective, 126
  contemporary views, 127, 128